The Seven Jewels of Reiki

By Sifu Michael Fuchs

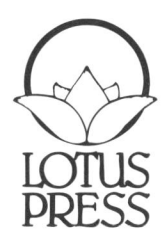

LOTUS PRESS

©2020 By Sifu Michael Fuchs

ALL RIGHTS RESERVED. No part of this book may be reproduced in any form or by any electronic or mechanical means including information storage and retrieval systems without permission in writing from the publisher, except by a receiver who may quote brief passages in a review.

First Edition 2020

ISBN: 978-1-6086-9247-7

Library of Congress Number: 2020930769

Published by:

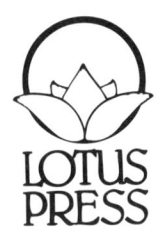

LOTUS PRESS

Lotus Press
P.O. Box 325
Twin Lakes, WI 53181 USA

800-824-6396 (toll free order phone)
262-889-8561 (office phone)
262-889-2461 (office fax)

www.lotuspress.com (website)
lotuspress@lotuspress.com

Printed In USA

DEDICATION

Humbly, I dedicate this book to:

The Universal Life Force,
which creates, nurtures, and sustains All,
and without which all Light would be extinguished, forever.
Namaste.

My beloved Mother,
whose selfless love through very dark, painful,
and trying times has allowed me to live, learn and grow.
Thank you Mom, I love you.

My amazing and wonderful teachers, mentors and guides.
Thanks for putting up with me.

Proudly, I carry your energy and legacy forward. *Namaste.*

FOREWORD BY DR. ETHA BEHRMANN

Michael's "The Seven Jewels of Reiki" showcases his path to reiki from initial skepticism to compassion and love of the art. You are led in a gentle way to follow his discovery and astonishment, with many anecdotes and stories, to relate to a rather simple and yet seemingly complicated topic. Michael does well to put the "I can't tell you, but I can show you," in conversational-style book form. You may as well be sitting at a fireplace listening to him tell his story. As you listen and gain more understanding of the art through the many comparisons, everyday ideas and situations, you gain a deeper understanding and are brought back to the true and pure elements, traditions and essence of reiki in modern day terms. Here you have a teacher who understands how easy learning can be if you keep a light and compassionate touch through a conversation, rather than lecture. In my own teachings, I have come to cherish the moment when students walk away thinking they had known most of what I taught them before; I know then that I succeeded in teaching them with ease, rather than being disappointed that I could not amaze them with my knowledge, which is now theirs.

I invite you to touch Michael's Butterfly Reiki System, hold it gently and then let it free. This book will be a fun addition to any reader's library, novice or experienced alike.

Etha Behrmann, *Ph.D. Physiology & Neuroscience*
MELT instructor

Etha teaches people of all ages and abilities how to relieve pain and disabilities by rehydrating their connective tissues with the MELT method as well as increasing performance by readjusting their nervous systems for a better and more effective, strong and pain-free body.

Current residence: P.O. Box 519, High Rolls, NM 88325

Website: http://www.sacramentochi.com
Email: etha@sacramentochi.com
Facebook: https://www.facebook.com/MELTwithEtha/

PREFACE

"Dream."

-the final teaching of Zen Master Takuan

Well hello there, it's a pleasure to meet you. It's no accident that this book is in your hands, as the Universal Life Force brings us all together. This is one of the most simple, yet profound truths we come to realize through receiving the blessings of the compassionate healing art of reiki. Namely, ALL IS ONE, WE ARE ONE. The same perfect and pure, eternal and indestructible pulsing cosmic life force which flows through me also flows through you. And indeed, flows through us all; as well as all of manifest and un manifest creation. This magnificent force has had many names throughout human history. Those of us who are practitioners of Usui Reiki Ryoho usually refer to it as reiki ("ray-key"), or in English, simply as the Universal Life Force. Another truth, which we must understand, is that She is truly beyond all names and transcends all dogmas or teachings- more on that later.

The intent of this book is two-fold: 1.) To present the fundamentals of the art of Usui Reiki Ryoho in a more complete and comprehensive fashion than is usually seen, and 2.) To unveil my own unique presentation of Usui Reiki Ryoho, which is known as the Butterfly Reiki System (BRS). BRS is an integrated reiki system modeled upon traditional Usui Reiki Ryoho as taught by the founder of the art, O-Sensei Mikao Usui, and his immediate disciples and heirs. It is composed of various well-known, as well as highly unique elements. These are drawn from my over thirty years of formal study and experience with reiki and related arts.

Overall it is my goal that this art be recognized as the great art that it indeed is; and that it takes its rightful place alongside the other wonderful and traditional Asian meditative, martial and healing arts - arts such as yoga in all of her manifestations: ch'i gung (qigong), t'ai chi ch' uan (taiji quan), aikido, Asian body work, massage and medicine, Shaolin kung fu; and so many others. It is certainly deserving of this, due to its effectiveness, practicality, safety, popularity, and uniqueness. There is no other art like this one, and she is not a "here today, gone tomorrow" or "flash in the pan" type of art. Reiki is here to stay!

Despite the fact that I have at least tens of thousands of hours of formal study, practice, and teaching experience - including as a lineage disciple receiving very unusual and in-depth, comprehensive training - I do not consider myself to be a "Master of Reiki." This term has been so overly utilized, mis-utilized, and debased to the point that it is virtually useless, even worse than useless. It is completely misunderstood and negatively confusing to both the general public as well as to reiki students and teachers themselves. And please understand that I mean no disrespect to anyone, and I say this gently and with compassion. This is part of my intent and goal, that the art (including its terminology and methodology) more realistically and accurately reflect the traditional intent and teachings of the Founder.

In the end we are all just students of reiki, with some of us having the extra blessing to serve as teachers, guides or mentors (as a "Reiki Sensei"). That's it, plain and simple. For reiki Herself is the Master, and we are all Her humble students. It's very important that we reiki people keep our feet on the ground and the ego in check, as it has always been taught in the true Asian arts.

The actual process and journey of writing this book and getting published proceeded from simple and straightforward to quite challenging and circuitous. The simple part was the actual writing process. As I had taught so many thousands of reiki and related classes over the years, from 1 hour to day long and multi- day workshops / retreats in every conceivable environment, I knew the material inside and out. At a certain point around 2011 like many in that economy I found myself unemployed for the first time in my life. This situation persisted for three years including sleeping on the floor and being one small step from homeless, but that's another story for another day.

Being unemployed I made the best of the situation and in addition to looking for work each day I began expanding on the outline for a reiki healing arts textbook which I had begun some years earlier, which became the book you are now reading. Once I had a working outline I began writing. My typical writing sessions began each day between 3:00 a.m. and 5:00 a.m. and proceeded on average for 3-8 hours, virtually every day for three and a half months, at which point the book was finished. I began each day by editing the previous days writing, then I proceeded to write new material. As I wrote the book grew and transformed, like a living being growing from infancy to adulthood. I had virtually zero distractions and was able to devote myself to the writing process in a pure fashion.

I must give thanks to the Founder, O-Sensei Mikao Usui, for guiding me throughout the entire writing process and since then. I made specific use of special reiki meditations and invocations in order to be guided directly by Spirit and O-Sensei before beginning each writing session, in order that I would be able to write the very best book possible, for the Highest Good of

All, Thy Will Be Done, not mine. From moment one I not only felt O-Sensei's presence, I "saw" him and often felt as if I was enveloped in a nurturing and inspiring cocoon of violet reiki energy as I wrote. I must say it was an awesome and humbling experience, to literally have your "voice" and pen be guided by Higher Powers this way.

The circuitous part of the journey is everything that came next. I knew I had written a good book, and this was confirmed by several people who reviewed it for me. As I learned, however, having a quality product is only one part of the publishing puzzle. Publishers very, very rarely will publish a book by an author who does not have an agent. In fact, many publishers won't even accept a submission from an author without an agent. I was determined to try, however, and sent my book to dozens of publishers who might publish a book such as this over a period of years. I was turned down each and every time, usually gently and often with praise. I must especially thank the publisher of a very well known and high quality book publishing company who personally sent me a glowing review, calling my book an "important work" and praising my writing skills. This gave me confidence to hang in there until I was eventually introduced to my agent.

How that happened is its own wonderful bit of synchronicity. I had been online complaining about my situation - I knew I was sitting on a quality book and could write many more, and of diverse styles, but how was I going to get there? Once you find your "voice" writing becomes a virtually effortless endeavor- but still, you need the connections!

Well, the "Universe" heard my sincere entreaties and responded by sending me a human angel to assist. A martial artist who I was familiar with online but in fact had never met, contacted me "out of the blue" one day to tell me he was going to recommend me to his agent! This was a selfless act for which I will be forever grateful. It turned out to be a better connection than I could ever have imagined as my agent is a true professional with decades of experience who has represented N.Y. Times best-sellers, and he also has his own publishing coming. Voila, I was in business.

He wisely recommended we start with another book first as I had already been sending this one to publishers for years. This resulted in my first book, "The Shaolin Butterfly Style - Art of Transformation." Once that was set I went back to this one – eight years after writing it - pulling it all together, and editing and simplifying it a bit.

While writing this book and going through the journey to getting it published I was also undergoing a profound personal transformation, being subject to healing and transformational powers from within and without. This basically threw my already upside-down world into a cyclone like whirlwind. Even now eight years later I am still integrating all of this, but it is much smoother now, thankfully. Look up "kundalini awakening" to get an idea of what I am talking about, Gopi Krishna style - more on that in the future, perhaps.

There are so many I need to thank for their invaluable contributions towards making this book possible. First of all, my parents, especially my Mom, for giving me an artistic vision and appreciation right from birth.

Of course this book would not have been possible without the great leadership and teachings of my taiji and martial arts teacher. In addition to his pure and ultra-high-quality arts and curricula, he passed on to all of us, especially his disciples/Sifu, the true way of the arts, the Dao. In fact, he even gave me his name, which I proudly carry to this day - Dao Chan I. Dao is the lineage name of his branch of White Lotus Shaolin Five Form Fist, he is Tao Chi Li.

I must also thank all of the other tremendous martial arts/taiji/qigong/meditation/reiki/spiritual teachers I have also been blessed to learn from since birth. Like the facets of a beautiful jewel all has coalesced to form this book and the Butterfly Reiki System.

Great thanks to my first reiki teachers, Cynthia and John, for opening the Way of reiki for me. They are wonderful and sincere reiki teachers who learned in a direct line from Rev. Takata, to John Harvey Gray, to me. To my next reiki teacher and the one I did the bulk of my early reiki training with including being trained and attuned as a reiki teacher, many, many thanks. This is Susane, a most inspiring and gifted reiki teacher and true clairvoyant. You rock, lady!

Much appreciation and thanks to my third reiki teacher, the pioneer and leader Patricia. Pat is a teacher originally from the Takata styles that originally traveled out from Hawaii. Along the way on her reiki journey she encountered the rare reiki arts of Reiki Jin Kei Do and Buddho Enersense, of which she is now a leading teacher. She was very generous with me in sharing her knowledge and skills of reiki and these arts in particular. I look forward to one day finishing training with her in these arts.

Along the way I also networked with and learned from and exchanged with quite a few other reiki teachers in reiki arts as diverse as Essential Reiki, Japanese reiki styles, and everything and anything related to reiki that I could find. This included of course reading every book I could find on reiki and related arts.

This led me quite by accident to my most profound reiki teacher by far, the famous living legend Burmese grandmaster, Dr. Maung Gyi. At a clinic I attended in upstate New York on the Korean Conflict U.N. Baton System that Dr. Gyi was leading (he was an original U.N. Peacekeeper in this very first deployment of U.N. Peacekeepers, at that time they did not carry firearms) it became evident that not only was Dr. Gyi the most tremendous martial arts teacher that I had ever met, he was also in possession of rare knowledge and skills with Asian healing and meditative arts. He wove this knowledge into his teaching of the Korean Conflict baton techniques.

As my teacher had a connection to and knew Dr. Gyi going back to the early 1970's via his teacher the late great Dr. Daniel K. Pai (Dr. Pai and Dr. Gyi were good friends and peers), Dr. Gyi took a liking to me right off. I seized the opportunity and invited Dr. Gyi to teach at my school, which he accepted and directed me to disciples of his to set-up. I was lucky and blessed that he allowed me to pick the material he was going to teach. As I was already the beneficiary of world class martial arts training, I asked Dr. Gyi to teach us methods and material specifically designed to enhance our reiki healing arts knowledge and skills - whereupon, he generously led multiple day long and multi-day seminars on rare spiritual healing arts and methods from his Burmese lineages and from his vast knowledge in general. This also included personal training with Dr. Gyi during his visits over the years. He is very tireless and generous.

This rare reiki knowledge encompassed all aspects of reiki healing arts: hands-on methods, reiki meditation, principles and concepts, unique reiki-ko methods, unique reiki symbols and their uses from his ancient lineages, and more. Much of this material is contained in this book, what is relative to the novice/intermediate levels of my Butterfly Reiki System. Dr. Gyi was quite pleased and encouraged me when I showed him the beginnings of my work integrating the methods and knowledge he shared with me with my knowledge of Usui Reiki Ryoho, Usui Shiki Ryoho, and other Usui influenced reiki arts.

Again, being so kind and generous (and downright utterly hilarious!) he also specifically and personally empowered me to share what he had shared with me, "with everyone" as he put it; when he said this he touched his heart and made a gesture outwards, to the whole world. This was in the driveway of my student's house in West Hartford, quite a way to start the day. It has taken awhile but you are now reading the first major step in that process. Namaste and great thanks to you, Sir.

I must also thank the pied-piper of reiki, Mr. Walter Luebeck of Germany for his wonderful inspiration and example as a leader and teacher of the art of reiki. We met end of July 2019 and had a wonderful visit and dinner. Hi Walter!

The final leg of the publishing journey for this book came in the late Summer of 2019, when I was led to send the complete manuscript to Lotus Press, publishers of top quality books on reiki and holistic arts. They suggested I split the long, 500 page or so original book into two shorter, more manageable books. This was a great idea and simple to accomplish, as the original manuscript was composed of two sections, one on more general reiki information and the other on more technical concepts and methods of the art. So, after some re-shuffling and final editing, just like magic - shazam!- one book became two. These being "The Seven Jewels of Reiki" and "The Compassionate Touch of Reiki: Healing Concepts, Elements, Methods." Together these books are meant to support each other and serve as the foundation of the Butterfly Reiki System, as well as textbooks for any other style of Usui Reiki Ryoho.

Of course I must thank my two wonderful editorial assistants, Christina DiTomasso and Nicole Updegrove: as well as Bob and Beth at Pronto Printer in Newington, CT and Daschle at Prentis Printer in Meriden, CT. Without their technical skills this book would not have been possible. Thanks all!

May the blessings be,

Michael Fuchs

Preface begun in June, 2013, New Britain, CT and finished in Spring, Summer and Fall in Rocky Hill and West Hartford, CT in 2019.

TABLE OF CONTENTS

Dedication III

Foreword by Dr. Etha Behrmann V

Preface VII

CHAPTER ONE: *Essential Reiki Foundations*

Essential Reiki Foundations 3

What is Reiki? 5

What is Usui Reiki Ryoho? 11

The Scope of Reiki Healing 17

    Reiki Meditation 18

    Reiki Energy Healing 19

    Reiki Spiritual Healing 26

How Does Reiki Work? 31

    What is the Reiki Attunement? 33

The Place of the Ego in Reiki 35

General Principles and Concepts of Reiki 39

What is the Butterfly Reiki System? 51

What Makes a Butterfly? 57

Why Reiki? 61

    Summary of Chapter One: 64

CHAPTER TWO: *The Seven Jewels of Reiki*

The Seven Jewels of Reiki 67

The Seven Jewels of Reiki Overview 69

    Gassho 71

    Reiju 73

Gokai	82
Reiki-ko	91
Jumon	103
Shirushi	108
Reiki Chiryo-ho	110
Summary of Chapter Two:	120
Appendix: Reiki Historical Documents	121
Reiho Choso Usui Sensei Kudoku No Hi	123
Questions & Answers From The "Hikkei"	127
Mrs Takata and Reiki Power	133
An Interview With Takata-Sensei, May 17, 1975	135
Author's Biography	139

CHAPTER ONE:
Essential Reiki Foundations

"In theory, practice and theory are the same.
But in practice, they are not."

-Yogi Berra, wise baseball guru

What is Reiki?

Quite simply, reiki is the compassionate touch of the love and grace of the Universal Life Force. There really isn't much more that needs to be said. But of course we do need to say so much more, as we adults often come to reiki with many blocks in our minds and hearts, and much negative pre-conditioning. Keep in mind though, that no words can truly convey the experience and the profound power of this perfect energy and great art. Like music or painting, how can one with mere words convey to one who cannot see or hear, their beauty? Truly "a picture is worth a thousand words." It is the same with reiki, and more so - the experience is virtually indescribable. However, in this book I have striven to paint a beautiful "reiki portrait" for you. As the Universal Life Force Herself has guided my pen and empowered my voice, I hope that you find the results illuminating and enjoyable.

I find that children often make the best reiki practitioners, as generally their minds and hearts are much more open and in tune: to themselves, to Nature, to other people, and to the Universe in general. I'll never forget the first time I taught and attuned a child to reiki. His Mother was a reiki student of mine, and naturally she began giving her son reiki. He was an intelligent young lad of about eight years old. Well, as often happens, he enjoyed the reiki so much that he told his mom that he wanted to learn. And he was quite insistent about this request. She wasn't so sure about this, however, and called me to ask me about it, whereupon I told her that of course he could learn. So we set up a children's version of a reiki class, which basically consists of me giving the child the simplest of instructions, asking if he or she has any questions, and then providing and facilitating the "reiki attunement." After this, the parent guides the child regarding reiki, with my consultation as needed. So I gave this enthusiastic young fellow the reiki attunement, which he loved, and asked him if he had any further questions. His astounding reply was, "Nope, I already know what to do."

Ah, another example of how much children can teach us, and of how much we could learn by becoming in so many ways more "child-like." Not every reiki class is this simple, I can assure you of that! Afterward, his mom reported that immediately after receiving his reiki attunement, her son began sharing reiki with other children that he felt would benefit from or enjoy it, in school and in his neighborhood. A budding young saint this boy was. This beautiful and blessed reiki lesson touched my heart and made me feel like a proud reiki grandpa.

In this book I am attempting to convey the art and the concepts of this art in as simple yet comprehensive a way as possible. This way it can be of benefit to the widest audience: those who have never heard of reiki; those who are interested in reiki and want to learn more; and of course those who are already reiki practitioners or teachers. So this book has been designed as an introduction to the foundational and essential methods and concepts of the art, and as a guidebook for reiki students. Keeping this in mind I must mention, however, that practicing the art daily is much more important and valuable than reading and contemplating the theories and concepts which underlay it. Practice and experience with reiki is more important than theory and intellectual knowledge of reiki - just as eating nutritious food every day is obviously preferable to reading and thinking about it! This is especially important for those new to reiki to understand - She is a completely experimental art and a highly compassionate one; rather than a technical and coldly intellectualized one. The most important aspect of learning properly is having an experienced, sincere, and compassionate reiki guide or sensei. Eventually reiki Herself may guide us, but until then a humble yet proficient living mentor is so helpful.

So reiki is the compassionate touch of the love and grace of the Universal Life Force. But what does this mean? Well, it can mean many things, such as:

- Reiki is a perfect and pure, timeless and eternal, healing energy/force.
- Reiki does not discriminate, and operates beyond all names, dogma, or teachings - as we are all beloved and equal sons and daughters of the same Universal Life Force in Her eyes.
- Reiki provides nourishment, support, healing, and positive transformation and empowerment for all beings and all of manifest and un-manifest creation.

At this point I want to emphasize that neither reiki as a healing force, nor the healing art of reiki (Usui Reiki Ryoho) are religious or faith healing arts or concepts. All people, whatever their belief system may be (or lack of one), can benefit from and make positive use of this energy and of this art, freely and with no strings attached This includes atheists, agnostics and scientifically-minded people, as well as people of all religious and spiritual beliefs. I know this is a fact in my mind, heart and soul - as well as from my experience of having taught and empowering hundreds of people of all manners of religious, spiritual, and agnostic/atheistic belief systems. This includes Priests, Nuns, Ministers, Monks,

CHAPTER ONE: Essential Reiki Foundations

and Wiccan High Priestesses ("good" witches), as well as so many others: truck drivers, welders, housewives, doctors and nurses, I.T. pros and technicians, children, seniors, the disabled, homeless, prison populations, and more.

Reiki blesses and benefits us all! For those who are atheistic or scientifically minded, reiki may be thought of as "natural, scientific, universal, healing energy." For those with specific religious or spiritual beliefs, each of us can conceive of reiki depending upon the teachings we know and accept. It's like how we can all appreciate and benefit from dentistry, despite what our various dogmas may be. Or like how we can all benefit from food, Reiki is freely available to all, just as these others are - no strings attached.

Quite simply, we may believe that reiki is a natural healing energy which exists in the universe (like untold numbers of other energies), or we may believe that reiki comes from God or whatever our concept of the Deity or the Divine is, or we may believe some combination of these two. Personally, I believe that both are true, and that science and spirituality are not in conflict. In fact, they are merely two different approaches with different "faces," but they are attempting to discover and elucidate the same things. However, I strive to present the essence of the art and to share its vital elements, concepts, and methods in as universal a fashion as possible. The rest, whatever you believe, is up to you.

The founder of this great and compassionate art, O-Sensei Mikao Usui, purposefully did not create a religion with a strict and rigid dogma. He wanted his revelations and teachings to benefit as many people as possible, and he accepted all people of good intent as students. Plain and simple, reiki is for everyone. If we adults could only approach the art as little children do, we would intuitively understand and accept this and know just what to do, as my first child reiki student knew and taught me.

The Seven Jewels of Reiki

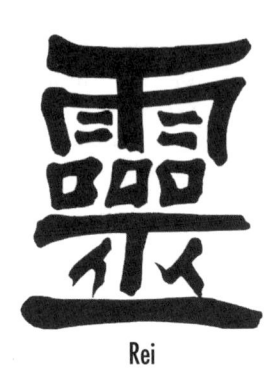

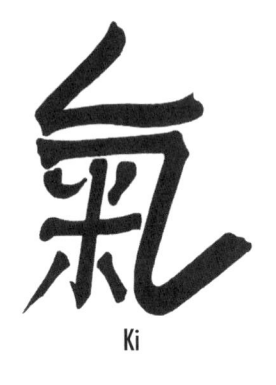

Rei

Ki

These are the traditional kanji characters (ancient Chinese writing) for the word reiki. Reiki may be translated from the ancient kanji to English in a number of ways. The top character, rei, refers to the higher, perfect, pure and eternal energy, dimension or universe. The bottom character, ki or (ch'i/qi), refers to the life-force, the energy of life, or the energy of our universe and all beings. When they are put together like this to form the characters and the word "reiki" they result in various possible definitions.

Here are some of the possible translations of the reiki kanji characters:
- The Universal Life Force
- Soul Power
- Divine Healing Energy
- Pure Realm Healing Energy
- Spiritual Healing Force
- God's Healing Light
- Spirit Gives Life (this is my favorite one)

Reverend Hawayo Takata, the woman primarily responsible for transmitting O-Sensei Usui's great art to the world beyond Japan, referred to reiki as "God Power," amongst other similar descriptions. Concepts similar to reiki have been taught and accepted in many cultures and all over the world since before the beginning of recorded human history. Although the art of reiki - Usui Reiki Ryoho - is quite modem and completely unique (O-Sensei passed on in 1926), as I say, reiki and similar concepts and terms are ancient. These include the "divine light," the "maha-para-shakti," and "ling ch'i" (lingqi). If we think of the sun in our solar system as the source of reiki (the "divine") then the light, heat, and other energies she shares with us are the reiki (or, the "divine light").

The term "maha-para-shakti" is a Sanskrit concept from ancient India which refers to the "highest, greatest, most perfect and pure universal energy." This energy is eternal and non-dualistic; it is no less than God's perfect love, intelligence, and power personified and alive, which gives birth to all.

"Ling Ch'i" is essentially the Chinese way of saying reiki (or vice-versa as the kanji characters and concepts originated in China before Japan adopted them). It refers to the highest and purest energy available to a human being.

CHAPTER ONE: Essential Reiki Foundations

As Dr. Daniel Reid describes in his most recommended and wonderful book, "A Complete Guide to the Principles and Practice of Chi-Gung," "Ling-chi (spiritual energy) is the subtlest and most highly refined of all the energies in the human system."

Those who have taken to translating reiki into English as "ancestral spirits" are doing so out of a fixed understanding and mistaken view of some of the underlying religious, spiritual and cultural beliefs, in my humble opinion. The kanji characters for the word reiki can indeed be translated into English in various ways. But the vast majority of reiki people are practicing the art-and conceive of it as an art of healing and of living - non-denominational, universal, and practical - not as rigidly dogmatic teachings. Now, if you seek to practice and conceive of the art as a Taoist, Shinto, Buddhist, or religious art, or anything like that, then perhaps you might want to use a translation of reiki that fits your particular religious beliefs and teachings. Otherwise, the translations should reflect reiki as a pure energy of healing - as we are presenting and utilizing the art as a spiritual, energetic healing art, not a religion.

What makes the art of Usui Reiki Ryoho unique is that it offers a shortcut to achieving, developing and working with this blessed celestial energy (but it's not a short-cut to mastery, this only comes the old-fashioned way); compared to traditional yogic, ch'i gung, or other similar traditional and ancient spiritual/energetic arts. This was the great gift and blessing which the universe bestowed upon O-Sensei Usui: a simplified but pure and powerful method which all people could easily learn and practice. In the past (before O-Sensei) only the most disciplined, talented, and advanced Yogis, Ch'i-Gung Masters, Monks, Saints, and Sages could achieve something like reiki healing ability. Thanks to the ultimate compassion of the Universe and of O-Sensei Usui, the path is open to all now. With the greatest and highest respect and gratitude I bow to them - Namaste!

Let me finish this sub-section with a quote from the H.H. Sant Kirpal Singh: "We have an Upanishadic text that tells us that Truth is one, though sages have described it variously. But to define IT is to limit, and since Truth (i.e. the whole Truth) is illimitable, IT, by Its very nature, remains undefined. It is more a matter of inner experience and realization than of comprehension and apprehension on the intellectual level." [1]

---

[1] For an in-depth and fascinating presentation on the many facets and aspects of this cross-cultural and interfaith phenomenon, I would direct the interested reader to the classic work by the great sage H.H. SantKirpal Singh *Naam or Word*.

What is Usui Reiki Ryoho?

"Our method is something completely original, there is nothing like it in the whole world Therefore, I want to share it with the public for the benefit of all humanity. Everyone has the potential to receive the spiritual gift, uniting body and soul, a divine blessing. Our method is an original one, based on the spiritual power of the universe. By this power, first a person becomes healthy, then the mind becomes calm and life becomes more joyous."

- O-Sensei Mikao Usui

So spoke the founder of this art, O-Sensei Mikao Usui (1865-1926), close to one hundred years ago now. His words are as true today as they were then. O-Sensei Usui was a great and highly accomplished and compassionate Saint and Avatar from Japan, whose art and teachings have positively impacted many millions of people the world over, and in a short period of time. O-Sensei was a rare blend of a mystic explorer of human and universal consciousness, combined with a visionary yet practical-minded teacher and leader. He straddled and mastered the ancient and modern worlds of his time. Via a powerful enlightenment experience and Universal Reiki Attunement on sacred Mount Kurama, which bestowed upon him the gifts of reiki and self-realization, he developed his art in the turbulent era after the turn of the nineteenth century in Japan. O-Sensei is more commonly referred to as either Dr. Usui or as Master Usui. I prefer to utilize some of the Japanese terms and titles for various key aspects of reiki and the art of reiki, as they give a more accurate description of the concepts being described. "O-Sensei" is a rare traditional title, which means something like "great, most high and special

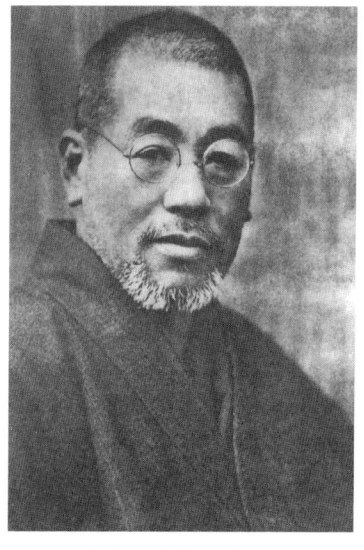

O-Sensei Mikao Usui

guide, teacher and mentor." O-Sensei is to sensei as Superman is to man, in other words. It designates one as a truly remarkable practitioner and leader. It is generally reserved for the most highly developed and unusually gifted Founding Grandmasters, such as O-Sensei Usui, or a younger contemporary of his, the famous Founder of Aikido ("The Way of Harmony"), O-Sensei Morihei Ueshiba. Note how this title, O-Sensei, gives a much different and more accurate description of what and who O-Sensei Usui was and is, compared to the rather mundane (but certainly respected) titles of Doctor or Master.

The focus of this book is not so much on the history of reiki and of Usui Reiki Ryoho. That history, as best as we currently understand it, has already been shared and is easily available (see www.aetw.org). I am more focused on presenting the art in as comprehensive and practical a fashion as possible, as a compassionate art of healing for all people.

Other than this, the history and energy of the art is woven into the entire book as a whole, in a distilled seed essence, pure form. Thanks be to the Universal Life Force for guiding my pen and empowering my voice.

臼
井
霊
氣
療
法

Usui Reiki Ryoho

Like the term "reiki", Usui Reiki Ryoho may be translated in various ways, such as:

- Usui's Reiki Healing Art
- Usui's Universal Life Force Healing Art
- Usui's Spiritual Healing Method
- Usui's Art of Divine Light Healing

Quite simply, it became named after him, as he was the Founder of a unique art and path. As for O-Sensei, he generally just referred to it as "my method"; or more formally as his "method for achieving personal perfection." Keep in mind that while O-Sensei offered his art freely as a gift for all humanity (which was - and is - quite rare), this does not mean that he was keen on marketing and selling it as the latest, greatest "spiritual/energetic healing product" out there - like the newest and best toaster - quite the contrary, actually. My personal experience dealing with some of these rare individuals, and research shows, that the true Founding Grandmasters (such as O-Sensei Usui) are an unusual blend of ancient and modern, traditional and revolutionary. What they are most concerned with is passing on their art - its principles, concepts and methods - in as true and pure a way as possible to well-intentioned people. That's

CHAPTER ONE: Essential Reiki Foundations

it. "Branding, packaging, and marketing" are not part of their equation; not much anyway, if they are the real thing.

So, as O-Sensei Usui stated in the quote at the beginning of this section, while it is indeed true that his art is unique and incomparable, it is also true that he was not concerned with trifles such as coming up with a snazzy name to help "market" his art. Presumably, the term "Usui Reiki Ryoho" was coined by some of his students and disciples who carried on his work.

In the next chapter, The Seven Jewels of Reiki, we will begin to explore the core elements of O-Sensei's art, illustrating clearly just what it is composed of. For now I would like to introduce two other individuals who were vital to the history and development of Usui Reiki Ryoho.

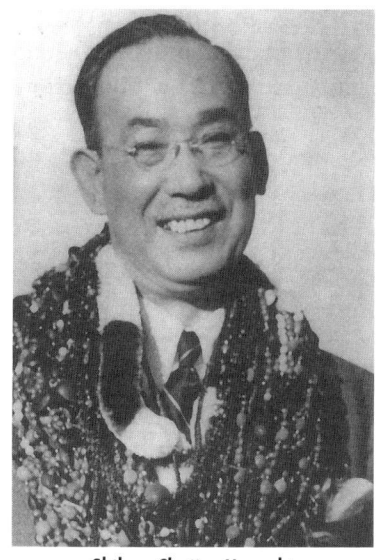

Shihan Chujiro Hayashi was a naval officer who was one of O-Sensei's most notable disciples. Disciples in an art like this are traditionally the few, rare individuals who due to their outstanding discipline, talent, perseverance, and character are chosen and earn the right to assist the head of the system (either the Founder or the current Headmaster) in preserving and passing on the art to the next generation. They are the fully empowered Teachers (Shihan) of the art, those whom the Founder/Headmaster has confidence in assisting him (or her) and those who essentially act as ambassadors and Ph.D. professors of the art. So, becoming a teacher in a traditional system (as O-Sensei taught and carried on the tradition) was not as simple as it is today. It was and is where this system of teaching and learning is still preserved, closer to the system utilized by quality schools of higher educations. In other words, just because you pay doesn't mean you pass. And just because you pass doesn't mean you get the Master's Degree, or much less a Ph.D. This would require much more than just "paying and passing"- more on that later.

Shihan Chujiro Hayashi

Shihan Chujiro Hayashi is notable regarding the history of Usui Reiki Ryoho for more than being one of O-Sensei's disciples, however. As a naval officer and a modern person for his time he was able to make some important innovations to the art, which made it more accessible to "regular" people. He utilized "reiki tables" (rather than sitting or lying on the ground) and opened "reiki clinics" and developed the modern style of reiki attunement, a version of which is utilized by the majority of reiki teachers now. He is also noted as being the teacher of Reverend Hawayo Takata, the lady primarily responsible for transmitting the art of reiki to the world beyond Japan; more on her in a bit. And we must also recognize (and never forget) his supreme example of ultimate compassion and self-sacrifice, his complete devotion to his art, and to his family. Rather than violate the teachings of his art and endanger his family, he refused the call to arms when his country infamously became involved with Hitler and WWII. However, simply refusing to go to war was not an option for him at this time in Japanese history, and would have brought great shame, misfortune, and punishment to his family for generations. The only acceptable option open to him for refusing to be involved in his country's obviously unjust military action, which would both protect his family and preserve his principles, was to commit ritual suicide (seppuku) in the manner of the ancient Samurai. Tears come to my eyes when I contemplate this: his awful decision and lack of good choices, and his ultimate compassion, courage, and honor. To those who do not respect Shihan Hayashi or hold him in low regard for some reason (maybe they don't like the military), I would encourage you to re-evaluate your thinking. Who amongst us - now or then - would have both the courage and the compassion to do this? This act of supreme self-sacrifice proves beyond a shadow of a doubt his high achievement as a great teacher of reiki. As far as I am concerned, he has entered the Sainthood for all time, just as his teacher did before him - great and most high Namaste to you, sir.

Reverend Takata is the individual primarily responsible for transmitting the art to the outside world. Her story is a truly remarkable one. She was born in Hawaii in the year 1900, for all intents and purposes as a slave (she was an indentured servant who worked on various farms).

Keep in mind that Hawaii did not become the 50th and final state of the United States of America until 1959. Back in 1900 it was an exotic and wild territory.

At a certain point in her life, being gravely ill and beaten down (but not broken!) by illness and misfortune after misfortune, she traveled to Japan to be with her family (her

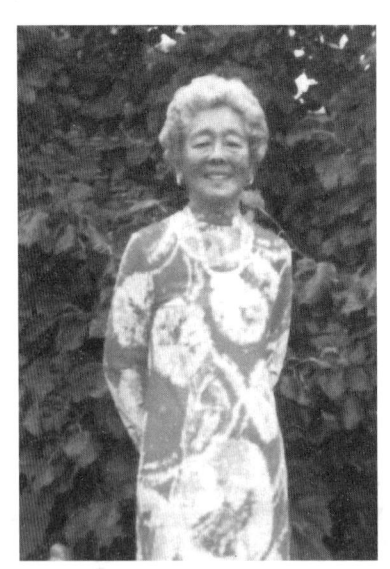

Rev. Hawayo Takata

parents had returned to their homeland) and received medical treatment. Quite simply, she was a mess, mentally and physically (her story is well-documented in great detail, it's a wonder she even survived). While in Japan seeking medical treatment, fate guided her to Shihan Hayashi and his reiki clinic. After only a few months of receiving regular reiki healing sessions she was completely whole again: in spirit, mind, and body. Considering this to be virtually miraculous, and being highly compassionate by nature, she wanted to become a reiki practitioner herself.

Although it was highly unusual at the time for him to do this as she was not a natural born Japanese citizen, Shihan Hayashi consented to her request. Shihan Hayashi, like his teacher, was also a visionary. He knew a great war was coming, and felt it important that this "foreigner" be taught, in order that she might preserve the art in case of disaster. How prophetic his decision turned out to be. Reverend Takata's "payment" for being given this great gift was that she was required to work in his reiki clinic for one year. After being accepted into the higher level of Okuden she returned home to Hawaii, taking the art with her. After proving herself through her continued discipline and sincerity, combined with her talent, in 1938 Shihan Hayashi traveled to Hawaii and empowered her as a fully trained teacher and disciple (Shinpiden), and assisted her in getting established in her practice of reiki in Hawaii. After his passing she became his heir and carried on his work.

Eventually Reverend Takata (she was a Minster in a spiritualist church) began taking and training her own disciplines in Hawaii as well as on the mainland U.S.A. and Canada. It is her disciples and their students who then brought this great compassionate art to the entire world. Thus she is really like the Reiki Mother of all reiki people, and should be greatly respected for this. I am in awe of what she was able to accomplish, given the extreme challenges she was faced with from birth. Reverend Takata passed on in 1980, but like O-Sensei Usui and her teacher Shihan Hayashi, her legacy lives on in many millions of reiki people now (and me!).

The Scope of Reiki Healing

"Meditation in various forms is practiced to achieve inner peace and tranquility, facilitate emotional and physical healing, generate internal energy, attain a higher state of consciousness or enlightenment, and/or to commune with the divine."

- Dr. M. Gyi

As a compassionate art of healing Usui Reiki Ryoho is both simple and profound. She positively impacts all aspects of an individual, as the following diagram illustrates:

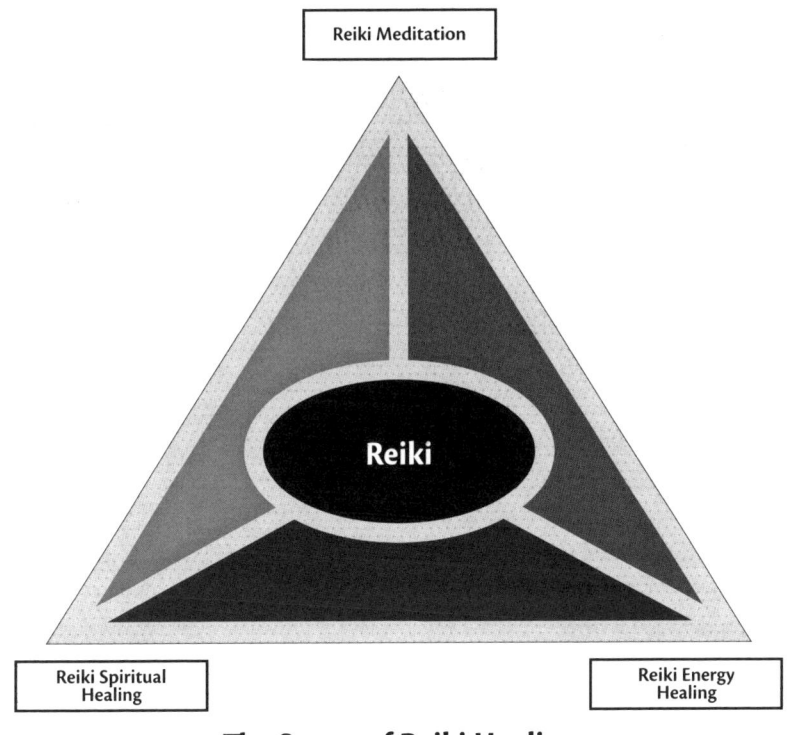

```
            Reiki Meditation

                  /\
                 /  \
                /    \
               / Reiki \
              /_____\

Reiki Spiritual              Reiki Energy
   Healing                      Healing
```

The Scope of Reiki Healing

The Seven Jewels of Reiki

In the next chapter we will discuss the seven core elements of Usui Reiki Ryoho ('The Seven Jewels'). For an in-depth discussion of the concepts, elements, and methods of these seven jewels see my book "The Compassionate Touch of Reiki: Healing Concepts, Elements, Methods. The diagram on page 17 illustrates in a more general and simplified fashion the overall scope, height, depth, and breadth of the art, as it was developed and taught by O-Sensei and his disciples.

Let's explore these three interconnected aspects of Usui Reiki Ryoho:

Reiki Meditation

Reiki Meditation can be quite diverse, and may involve any and all aspects mentioned in the quote at the beginning of this sub-section (Dr. Gyi is one of the Western world's great pioneers and leaders of Asian martial, meditative, and healing arts. Originally from Burma, he settled in the United States after World War II. He is also - by a very wide margin - the most skilled and knowledgeable reiki teacher that I have been blessed to learn from).

Reiki meditation is the essential glue that holds the entire art together and allows for reiki skills and healing abilities to be further developed. Reiki meditation also includes character developing methods and aspects, such as: reverence for life, non-violence, universal love and compassion for self and all, forgiveness, and more. Reiki meditation also encompasses various breathing, reiki generation, and reiki circulation and transmission methods (reiki-ko), as well as encompassing reiki skill building and sensing aspects of the art (byosen reikan-ho and reiji-ho). Additionally, reiki meditation is essential to the healing and transformative aspects of the art (reiki energy healing and spiritual healing).

Thus, reiki meditation is the bedrock foundation from which all reiki seeds, roots, trunks, branches, leaves, flowers, and fruits depend upon and develop from.

While it is indeed true that Usui Reiki Ryoho is quite unique in that virtually all people can easily, simply, and safely learn and practice the art right from the moment after receiving a reiki attunement (and often with excellent results) - it is also true that reiki meditation allows for greater enjoyment and a deeper experience, especially in regards to the possibility of long-term growth and healing as a reiki practitioner and as an individual. It helps to keep the reiki path focused for us, as well as in discovering new reiki paths that we may travel.

Imagine reiki meditation like a universal G.P.S. system combined with a cosmic computer and internet hookup, all contained within our very own starship (us) - the possibilities are endless!

And how much and how often should one practice reiki meditation? I will pass on to you the advice my t'ai chi teacher gave to me when I asked him the same question (adapted to reiki): think of reiki meditation like food. A little every day is much preferable to a lot once a week! Now go, enjoy some peaceful and healing reiki meditation.

Reiki Energy Healing

This is the aspect of Usui Reiki Ryoho that is most emphasized nowadays. In fact, the terms "reiki" and "energy healing" are often (erroneously!) utilized interchangeably. As if a meal in a five star, fine dining Italian restaurant is the same thing as lunch at a local McJunkFood outlet.

Reiki energy healing is indeed one of the main elements of the art, and to our great benefit for balance of mind and body. However, Usui Reiki Ryoho is a deep and well-rounded art, there is much more to it than energy healing alone.

The energy healing aspect of the art refers to utilizing reiki to cleanse and heal energetic blocks and imbalances at all levels of being: physical, emotional, mental, and at the soul level (or Higher Self if you prefer that term). Generally this happens at various levels of being simultaneously. This is why we always offer reiki for the Highest Good, Thy Will Be Done, not mine; rather than merely to address symptoms such as stress or pain. When reiki is utilized primarily for soul level healing, we are crossing over to the spiritual healing aspect of the art, which we will discuss next.

So, the reiki person may put her hands on her sore knee in order to get some pain relief from minor arthritis. The reiki may aid in relieving the pain, but at the same time her breathing may deepen, she may relax and become very calm, and she may receive insights into why her knees are sore. This may happen all at once, so as you can see, the compassionate art of reiki is so much more than a simple energetic bandage with which we patch up our blown energetic tires with! Witness O-Sensei's answer in the Reiki Ryoho Hikkei to the question, "Does Usui Reiki Ryoho cure diseases (physical) only?"

"No, not only cure diseases of the physical body but also mental illnesses i.e. anguish, weakness, cowardice, vacillation, nervousness, and other bad habits can be cured. And emphasis is placed on healing others with god-like or Buddha-like mind, and happiness can be mutually shared with others."

-Reiki Ryoho Hikkei, Hyakuten Inamoto translation

Note the last sentence of O-Sensei's answer, which points to the higher levels of the art and the possibilities contained within it. And I ask you: does an energetic aspirin or Band-Aid allow us to develop to a saintly level so that we may share true happiness with all? I don't think so. Not even the best soma can do that!

Let me share with you now some of the amazing and seemingly miraculous experiences which I and some of my students have had utilizing the reiki energy healing aspects of this great art:

- After took my very first reiki class (which was revelatory in nature and I am still processing) I began to right away practice on myself daily, with odd but enjoyable results. Well, after a couple of days it was time to go back to work as I had taken a few days off to fast, meditate, and fully let go into the reiki experience. At the time I was working in an acute care rehabilitation hospital, which like any hospital can be a stressful environment. Right off at 8:00 a.m. I went to see a friend of mine who also worked at the hospital, a martial arts buddy with whom I wanted to share my reiki experience. "John" had a big job at the hospital. He was in charge of all the graphic design, from the style of the letterheads on the official paperwork to the signs on the doors, the flashing lit-up words and logos on the outside of the hospital building, everything. It was a couple of weeks before Christmas and even though it was only 8:00 a.m., John already had a migraine headache. He had just gotten off the phone with the president and CEO of the hospital, who had been screaming at him to place a pair of gigantic, lit-up, Christmas trees on top of the hospital - and like now, yesterday if possible! And pronto, is it done yet? And no, I am not making this up. Forget the Christmas spirit, this guy "Dr. Romero" (the CEO) was more Capt. Ahab and Ebenezer Scrooge than Santa Clause, by many leaps of Santa's reindeer.

Well, seeing my friend in such a frazzled state of mind and already with a migraine headache, I offered to give him some reiki as I had just learned to do, and had been encouraged to share it with those in need. So John was

CHAPTER ONE: Essential Reiki Foundations

to be my first "reiki guinea pig!" Being good friends, he trusted me and was open to trying it. So I had him sit in his chair at his desk whilst I stood behind him, prepared myself, and gently and slowly lowered my reiki hands over his crown, as I had been taught.

After only a minute or two it felt as if my hands had literally melted into his skull. John was started to get so relaxed that he was melting, too. Then after a couple more minutes of this, there was literally a great flash of white light, and I backed up and removed my hands in bewilderment. John shook his head and asked me, "What was that?" We both weren't sure how or what had just happened - but his migraine headache was instantly gone!

-"Pete" was a kung fu student of mine who was suffering from severe insomnia - he had not slept more than fifteen minutes in over six months. One side of his face was perpetually clenched up like in a Bell's palsy or stroke victim, such was his intense stress level. After hearing that I was a reiki teacher and practitioner, and that reiki offers people great stress relief and relaxation, Pete approached me in desperate straits, "I'll try anything," he told me. Keep in mind that Pete had already been to many doctors and psychologists and tried many standard insomnia treatments and drugs, all to no avail. Many people come to reiki this way, as a last resort. Of course, reiki is best utilized for prevention and maintenance - rather than as intervention - which we shall explain later.

So on the appointed day and time Pete arrived for his reiki healing session. He laid down on the reiki table and I sat behind him near his head and prepared myself. Then slowly and gently, I placed my reiki hands over his crown. Within five minutes his whole body began shaking, vibrating, and convulsing like a giant Mexican jumping bean! Figuring his system was relieving vast amounts of stored tension, and being confident in the safety and power of reiki, I continued.

After a few minutes of this - Pete shaking and vibrating while I was giving him reiki - his head fell to the side and he began to snore loudly! He was taking very deep breaths, and snoring and snoring and snoring away. In fact, he slept throughout the entire hour-long reiki session, snoring blissfully. When I was done, I quietly left the room to call his wife and tell her what had happened, as I didn't want to wake him for his ride home - remember, he hadn't slept in six months. Ouch! His wife happily agreed to come get him, yelling over the phone, "No, don't wake him! Don't wake him! I will come and get him!"

She drove to our location and I literally carried Pete in my arms - he was still snoring, mind you, in a deep sleep - and poured him into the back seat of the car. When they got home, Pete's wife dragged him inside, and he slept for twelve hours straight.

Best of all - his insomnia was gone! For the six months that I knew Pete after this (until his work took him out of the country) he never had a problem sleeping again. Not bad for one $50 reiki session, eh? Reiki strikes again.

-"Alice" was a reiki student of mine, a nurse in her mid-fifties who took a level one reiki class (shoden) with me at a local community college. Like many nurses, she had heard of reiki, and wanted to take the class to see if it could help her twenty year-old daughter. You see her daughter was, umm, backed up, she had not been able to eliminate solid waste for months! Yes, nature's call for #2 was on a long and dreadful vacation. As with Pete, regular medicine wasn't helping so Alice figured she would give reiki a shot.

Alice took my class and during the course of training explained to me why she was there, and asked me when she could use reiki on her daughter. I told her that she could use reiki as soon as she got home, which she said she would do, as I taught her in class.

A few days later Alice e-mailed me with a report. She had gone home the night of the class and given her daughter a full body reiki session, focusing extra time on the abdominal region. She told me that soon after she was done her daughter went to the bathroom – and went, and went, and went some more! Nature had called, finally, and in a big way (as you can imagine after not being able to do this for months). Alice thanked me profusely for sharing this great gift with her and her daughter. Hallelujah for reiki!

-"Howard" was a reiki student of mine, a man in his forties. He took a reiki class with me at another local community college. As is the norm, at the beginning of the class we all took turns introducing ourselves and sharing any information we wanted, why we were there, questions we had, and the like. Now, as I have mentioned, for several years I worked in an acute care rehabilitation hospital. This included working daily with patients who had traumatic or acquired brain injuries. We had a lock-down TBI/ABI unit, and I would work with these people there or take them to other areas of the hospital. Now, I am no neuropsychologist or anything like this, I was a rehabilitation technician and primarily led therapeutic exercise routines for the various patients, amongst other activities. Still, people with brain injuries usually have some lingering symptoms, which someone used to working with this population can pick up; a slightly wandering or unfocused eye, an odd speech pattern, a wavering gaze, something.

Well, as Howard introduced himself and began to tell us his story, for all

CHAPTER ONE: Essential Reiki Foundations

intents and purposes he seemed to be in excellent health and in a completely "normal" condition for a man his age. He sure didn't seem to be a survivor of an extremely severe brain injury. But wait till you hear his story!

Howard began to share his story with us. About two years prior he was at a big summer family reunion and outdoor picnic. It was a large gathering and they organized a family softball game. Howard was playing left field, and his nephew in his twenties was at third base. Well, someone hit a high pop-up just outside the foul line and up past third base, in what is called no-man's land. Both Howard and his nephew took off simultaneously, running at full speed to try and catch the ball. Neither of them saw the other, as they were focused on the ball, and both dove head first to catch it. Well, they cracked heads in mid-air like rams during mating season. Not only was Howard knocked-out cold, he had suffered a brain injury, a terrible one. The brain injury had caused his senses, especially his visual and auditory ones, to be distorted and magnified, as if he was on a perpetual "bad LSD trip!"

Howard, a previously extremely fit and active man, had to sit day and night in a dark room with no noise, for many months. He told us that during this time a fly was like a loud buzzing helicopter and any light was like a kaleidoscope that made him nauseous and sick. Needless to say, Howard was extremely distressed about his situation, which seemed hopeless, and entered into a deep depression. He had gone from being a vibrant and healthy man in his prime, instantly, to being as far as he knew, permanently shut in a quiet, dark room - a horrible fate. Of course he was under all sorts of treatment, but nothing was helping.

Well, as fate would have it, one day his physical therapist - who was also a reiki practitioner - began to give him reiki. She did it out of boredom more than anything, as nothing else was helping him (she wasn't aware, obviously, of the power of reiki). Well, right away she noticed that it began to impact him positively. Seeing this, she began to give him full reiki healing sessions every week. After six months of this, amazingly, Howard's brain had healed itself - all of his symptoms were permanently gone! Howard told us that he now wanted to learn reiki so that he could share the art which had saved his life with others. What a great reiki blessing!

- "Jennifer" was quite an unusual woman. Yes, she was at Woodstock. And yes, she knew - and partied with - the "Black Panthers." She's been to Space Mountain (underlying Cheyenne Mountain, NORAD headquarters in Colorado), and has had quite a remarkable life. An extraordinary artist, she has done portraits for the likes of Vice President Al Gore, Polish President Lech

Walesa, and Great-Grandmaster Dr. Maung Gyi-and she's not even a portrait painter! She is the founder of the CT Plein Air Painting Society, her landscape paintings are beautiful and in demand. You might say her blood and soul carry the colors of the muse. She was born to create awesome works of art, and seemingly effortlessly, as the true artists do.

Unfortunately, as a young woman in her early twenties, Jennifer developed severe bleeding ulcerative colitis. And worse, there is no good medical treatment or cure for this awful disease. All the doctors could offer Jennifer was to try to help her manage her symptoms. For thirty years she suffered with this horrible affliction, she was close to death several times, and the disease took a terrible physical, emotional, mental, and spiritual toll upon her. At a certain point her doctor recommended she try taking some t'ai chi classes as a way to promote health and manage her stress. Good for you, doc! We need more open-minded physicians like this one. So this is how Jennifer and I met, while she was in desperate straits health-wise.

After she explained to me why she wanted to take t'ai chi lessons, I immediately suggested that she also try some reiki healing sessions. She agreed, and we set up a time for me to visit her in her home studio for her first reiki session (many more were to follow). Well, she enjoyed the reiki session very much, but it had a strange effect upon her - she didn't sleep for three days straight. Like most artists, Jennifer is very sensitive and her entire mind/body/energy system was completely imbalanced after thirty years of dealing with not only her illness, but also with the powerful medical shock treatments - drugs, drugs, and more drugs. So this first reiki session affected her deeply, kind of super-charging her at a deep level and preparing her for healing and re-balancing.

After three days of not sleeping she called me to ask me about it. I suggested she try another reiki session. Well, after this one, she basically slept for three days. After this her system began to balance itself, and she slept normally. At this point Jennifer decided to take reiki training from me in order to support her health through reiki self-healing on a daily basis. Keep in mind that she was also learning and practicing t'ai chi and wellness ch'i gung (qigong) daily.

Jennifer could feel right away that this potent healing trinity - reiki, t'ai chi, and wellness ch'i gung- was helping her, and she became quite disciplined about practicing daily - so much so that she actually became an instructor of both t'ai chi and reiki, and a fine one at that. I am very proud of her.

Well, after five years of this - daily reiki self-healing, regular reiki sessions which I gave her, as well as the t'ai chi and ch'i gung and a healthy diet - a

CHAPTER ONE: Essential Reiki Foundations

fateful day came when her doctor came out scratching his head after one of her regular visits. He told her, "Jennifer, whatever you are doing, keep doing it!" She was, and has stayed for years now, completely symptom free of the horrible curse which she had been afflicted with for over thirty years. The power of reiki had struck again! Jennifer is indeed a walking reiki miracle (and a piece of work). I couldn't resist that, hi Jennifer!

-"Esmeralda" is another amazing woman. She has been on a healing path since birth, constantly being tested by life in order that she might grow and evolve. And all the tests she has met and passed. She is very humble, but has seemingly endless talents. She is an artist, a singer and musician, a minister, and a powerful clairvoyant shamanic healer. She has actually worked successfully with the F.B.I. on numerous missing persons cases - think X-Files type of stuff, from her meditation room she goes into an altered state of consciousness and is guided to finding the missing people! She has a 100% success rate. She is a wonderful mother and wife, and another t'ai chi, reiki, ch'i gung student and instructor of mine. I am very humbled and blessed to have students such as this. Years ago she took a reiki class with me at a local community college, and being extremely organized and disciplined has gone on to study regularly with me, despite her busy schedule and home life. She is in such high demand as a shamanic healer that she is usually booked months in advance.

Sadly, her mother was recently diagnosed with a terminal lung cancer. Esmeralda's mother did not share her daughter's enthusiasm for the seemingly "strange and weird" healing arts, but due to her situation she agreed to allow her daughter to begin giving her intensive and daily hands-on and "distance" reiki healing sessions, along with utilizing her other healing gifts and talents.

Well, I think you know what is coming next. After a few weeks of this, Esmeralda's mom one day went in to see the doctor for a routine check-up and visit. He was not expecting there to be any positive changes as she had a terminal diagnosis. But he took x-rays of her lungs anyway. When they were developed, like Jennifer's doctor he could only scratch his head in wonderment, for the pictures and the tests had shown that the tumors had completely regressed – they were gone without a trace - another reiki "miracle." And even better, after receiving this great and blessed gift of a "second lease on life," Esmeralda tells me her mother had developed a much sunnier outlook on life, realizing that each and every day is indeed a sacred gift. Amen to this, and the power of reiki.

Please note that reiki does not take the place of standard medical or psychological care. Reiki is meant to be part of an overall wellness strategy and program, just as eating a healthy diet, daily exercise, and other good habits of mind and body are meant to be. That is it, plain and simple.

No worries, doc, we still need you - as you need us!

We will explore the concept and practice of reiki "distance" healing - what I refer to as Reiki Unity Healing - in great depth and detail in subsequent chapters and sections of this book.

Reiki Spiritual Healing

> "Our method is a spiritual one, it transcends medical science -it is not based on it."
>
> -O-Sensei Mikao Usui, Reiki Ryoho Hikkei[2]

Reiki spiritual healing refers to utilizing the art in order to unify the self with the Higher Self, or with the Soul, the Atman, the Great Spirit, God, Allah, the Buddha Nature, or whatever words you have for the perfect and pure, eternal higher dimension. It is essentially a higher form of reiki energy healing. In other words, inner healing of such great depth and power that personal transformation, evolution, and empowerment becomes a reality. This is no small feat, as it has been said that it is easier to move a mountain that it is to truly change ourselves. I was also taught that the only true miracle was a "permanent change to a higher level of consciousness." This is what reiki spiritual healing is all about.

Keep in mind that there is no end to this journey, no magic pot of gold at the end of the rainbow, which when achieved allows you to say, "Yay! I'm there now, let's go have a beer and celebrate!" There is no certificate or diploma for this either; and the only goal is this: the Path is the Goal. You must keep traveling this path, forever. And we each must travel our own path, no one else can do it for us or knows what is best for us. Only we do. But to know what it is we must learn to listen to the "guide within." When we embrace this consciously and surrender to it, we will begin to make progress. Good luck and may God bless you on your journey.

I once asked my Buddhist teacher, "What is enlightenment?" He was happy that I asked, and told me that he had asked his teacher the very same

---

2   James Deacon translation, www.aetw.org

CHAPTER ONE: Essential Reiki Foundations

question (his teacher is the famous and renowned Geshe Kelsang Gyatso). His teacher's answer was this: "Enlightenment is a state of consciousness that is all Light. A state of consciousness that contains no darkness, not even the shadows of the seeds of darkness - only pure spiritual Light." What a perfect answer! But far from easy to achieve, almost impossible actually; though we all have the potential to achieve this within us. In fact, this is the reason we are here, to achieve this and to lead others to it. Although I have been blessed to have had many enlightenment experiences, kundalini awakenings, out of body experiences, and other spiritual experiences since birth; alas, I have yet to enter this "blessed paradise" permanently.

But I have visited, and I can report that it is indeed a beautiful and marvelous place!

This same Buddhist teacher of mine was also an enthusiastic reiki practitioner and teacher. As an aside, he was English and from Liverpool and he had the exact same cockney accent as John Lennon. He was quite a riot to behold and listen to, as he sat on his throne with his bald head and saffron robes saying, "Right! We're all gonna meditate now!" like some reincarnated Buddhist version of an English rocker bad body... what a gem he was! He actually used to play bass guitar in rock and punk bands all over the U.K. and Europe.

He told me that he felt that the energy of reiki and the energy of Buddhism were one and the same. Interestingly, I have been told the same thing (but modified to their own beliefs/terminology) by Christian Priests, Ministers and Nuns; as well as by Hindus, Sikhs, Muslims, Wiccan High Priestess, Shamans and others. I know it to be true in my heart and soul, reiki does indeed appear to be none other than the pure essence of the Universal Life Force, above and beyond all dogma as reiki people all over the world can attest to. She is truly the Mystic Core, the Truth, the Love, the Light, and the Way. Amen.

Let me provide you with an example from my own experience of reiki spiritual healing:

- "Hank" was a kung fu student of mine, one of my very first students after I took over my teacher's school. Hank was about my age, and in fact, we had much in common regarding the painful lessons which life can teach from birth for some of us. I was a brand-new aspiring reiki teacher when I first got to know Hank, and had actually not taught or attuned anyone to reiki yet.

Knowing that Hank (who was a wonderful and sweet guy with a big smile) was homeless and attending A.A. and other self-help programs - in addition to being a fine and hard-working kung fu student of mine - I knew he could benefit from learning reiki. So I approached him and offered to teach him for free. I wanted a student to share reiki with so I could practice my new skills and he needed the reiki big-time - we were meant to find each other, it seemed.

We set up a time when Hank would visit to receive his reiki attunement and training, during which my school's other classes were not in session. Hank sat down whilst I began to perform the blessed ritual known as reiki attunement, which we will discuss in detail soon. He immediately - to my relief - could feel the reiki healing energy flowing through him and in his hands. Yay! It worked! So I then proceeded to teach him how to give himself reiki, share reiki with others, and the other elements of a basic reiki class.

This is where it gets interesting. Hank was quite disciplined in his goal to heal and improve himself. When he learned reiki he began to practice and give himself reiki daily. Like I mentioned, Hank had had a very hard life, which he was trying to put back together. In fact, just before I got to know him, his ex-wife had shut him out so strongly that she had actually gotten a court order which forbade him from seeing his children. Well, Hank loved his children and this - like the other tragedies, abuses, and traumas in his life - weighed very heavily upon him. Like many of us who have been traumatized and need to survive day-to-day, Hank was basically just blocking out and suppressing all of his pain and anguish, keeping it buried and hidden inside. He was just doing what he needed to do each day to get by, and in Hank's case, always with style and with a big smile.

So, Hank began daily reiki self-healing as part of his efforts to heal and improve himself. Well, the compassionate art of reiki can be very powerful at times. She is not a placebo nor is she a drug which masks pain. It ain't all roses, champagne, and chocolate on the reiki healing path, no siree! I know this one myself, all too well. All of the pain, anguish, and suffering which Hank had been suppressing came to the surface, at which point he actually became an outpatient of a psychiatric hospital. He was having flashbacks and couldn't control his emotions. Hank was undergoing a profound and rapid spiritual healing catharsis - which for those of us who have been there know, can almost feel worse than dying a tortuous death one minute, and then the roller coaster flips and you feel like you are the king of the world! And back and forth it goes.

Hank continued with his kung-fu training for a while with me, but eventually he moved on and I lost track of him. But I often thought of him, my first reiki student.

About a year later I happened to run into Hank on the street one day, to our mutual enjoyment, as like I said we had hit it off right from the beginning.

To my amazement and wonderment, he filled me in on what he had been up to and how his life had changed. Not only was he no longer homeless, he had an excellent full-time job and had met, fallen in love, and was living with a wonderful woman. Best of all, his ex-wife- no doubt seeing how much Hank had changed - had relented and was allowing him to visit and spend time with his children.

Hallelujah! All of this in one wild, roller coaster-like year.

As I drove off after talking to Hank that day I came to realize more than ever the great, awesome gift which the Universe had blessed me with. Wow! If reiki could help someone like Hank (or myself) in such a powerful way, what could it do for other, less-traumatized people? Hmmm, the sky is the limit...

So as you can see, reiki is indeed a true and powerful spiritual healing art. Keep in mind that while we are indeed all sons and daughters of the very same Universal Life Force, my path and your path will not be the same. There are many paths to the top of the mountain. To paraphrase Don Juan, whom Carlos Castaneda made famous, "All that matters is that we find a path with heart, one that resonates with us, and then to follow this path right to the very end." And keep in mind that what you seek is not to be found "out there" anywhere. As a great, high and perfect teacher said long ago, "Behold! The Kingdom of Heaven is within you." When you find your true self you will find this, as well. Namaste.

How Does Reiki Work?

"In every atom of this astounding universe, God is ceaselessly working miracles; yet obtuse man takes them for granted."

-Paramahansa Yogananda

The compassionate healing art of reiki is the most natural, safe, and effective art of its kind available. As we have mentioned, virtually all people can easily receive the gift of reiki healing ability. It is a part of our make-up as human beings, as a manifestation of our innate healing abilities. For instance, each month we regenerate a new stomach, so effortlessly that it is unnoticed. Even Jiffy Lube isn't this efficient! Mother Nature is the best every time.

One way to conceive of the Universal Life Force is to think of it as a kind of invisible super tonic/nutrient/vitamin/fuel - one which a human being is completely in resonance with. So when someone (or an animal, plant, or any being) receives reiki healing - whether from a reiki practitioner or in reiki self-healing for those who are reiki practitioners - the reiki is "digested" in a process which is very similar to digesting food. The main difference is that it is the individual's energy system which is absorbing, digesting, and making use of the reiki - rather than the physical digestive system (obviously).

The reiki is then utilized for the Highest Good of the individual, from the Soul or Higher Self level to the physical, and vice-versa. This happens quite naturally, in a way similar to how the nutrients from food are absorbed and utilized with no need for this process to be directed or controlled by us (luckily for us!). For you see, the reiki and the Soul or Higher Self are virtually one and the same, they are perfectly matched and conjoined genetic twins as it were. Matched and meant to be together in an eternal, blissful union.

This makes the process of reiki healing much simpler and safer than eating, actually. No chewing is required and no one is allergic to reiki!

The following are the main applications of reiki healing:
- Regeneration of spirit, mind, and body

- Maintenance of spirit, mind, and body
- Longevity of spirit, mind, and body
- Mental and emotional balance and harmony
- Spiritual clarity and tranquility
- Self-realization - personal transformation and attainment of Unity Consciousness

The first four of these are the basic applications of reiki healing, and are obtainable (depending on many factors) by most people with a modicum of self-discipline and creativity. The last two are the advanced applications of the art, theoretically obtainable by all, but rarely achieved perfectly in one lifetime.

While reiki is being studied by various medical and scientific organizations - as well as by the military and government (yikes!) - to date the exact manner in which reiki works and operates has not been scientifically ascertained. However, numerous "outcome based" studies have proven the effectiveness and safety of reiki.[3] So no worries, we don't know how gravity works either, but who would question its effectiveness?

Reiki and the art of reiki contribute greatly to relieving daily and accumulated stress, and enjoying life more. Thus, as described earlier, ideally this art is utilized in a preventative and maintenance fashion so that health, balance, and harmony for the total being may be achieved, maintained, and preserved. For the more serious and disciplined student, the art of reiki can be a life path. O-Sensei often referred to his art as his "method of achieving personal perfection."

It really shouldn't be thought of as an "energetic medical intervention" or as an exotic form of "energy medicine." The compassionate art of reiki was not designed nor intended to be this; though of course She may be applied as such (combined with standard medical care, if needed). The mind-set of reiki as "energy medicine" insults the art and teachings of O-Sensei, and greatly limits its scope and effectiveness. Ever hear of this one, "An ounce of prevention is better than a pound of cure?" We do preventative maintenance on our cars, this is exactly what Usui Reiki Ryoho is meant for, for us.

I like to think of the art of reiki – combined with a healthy diet, exercise, and related factors – as a human being's "owner's manual" for achieving and maintaining optimal wellness for mind and body. And just like the owner's manual for your car, no one should be without this vital "life manual" known as reiki. So get thee to a good reiki teacher, pronto!

---

[3]   See Hartford Hospital's website, Integrative Medicine Dept.

What is the Reiki Attunement?

The reiki attunement is the process and blessed ritual that transforms someone into a reiki practitioner. This is how one "learns reiki," as it were. Learning reiki is not so much a technical and intellectual process as it is a natural one. Though, of course, once attuned, people can and should study its concepts, methods, and applications, and practice to attain skills. But again, as previously mentioned, what is most important for reiki people is to make positive use of the art and energy of reiki daily. This is done via reiki self-healing, reiki meditation, and reiki-ko; as well as contemplating and living the principles, and sharing the art with others. We must strive each and every day to "Be Real, Be Reiki."

In the next chapter we will discuss the reiki attunement in great depth and detail. For now, let me describe it for you through a simple analogy. Imagine a building that has a power supply, as well as all of the necessary components to give light to the various rooms and areas of a building - from the basement and hallways all the way to the penthouse. Except there is one key item missing - the light bulbs! So, one could flip the switches on endlessly but not get the desired result. The potential for light to be there exists; it is just missing a key element for this to happen.

Well, during reiki attunement our personal "reiki light bulbs" are activated, so that naturally and effortlessly we can benefit from the Light (reiki) forever afterwards.

Another useful analogy is the radio. Radio waves existed long before the invention of the radio, ostensibly since the beginning of creation. We human beings, however, could not do much with them until the radio was invented. Regarding reiki and reiki attunement in this analogy: we are the radio, and the radio waves are like the reiki. And it is the reiki attunement which "tunes in" our "reiki channel" clearly and powerfully, so that we may benefit from her perfect celestial "programming" - forever! (God is the Radio Transmitter).

So in a way the reiki attunement is similar to a reiki healing session. Except the intent of all involved - the reiki student, the reiki teacher, and the reiki Herself - is for the student to be empowered with reiki healing ability. It is a natural process, like reiki healing is; as well as a natural function of the Universal Life Force and all living beings that this can happen. And thanks be to O-Sensei and the Universe for bringing the process of reiki attunement to the world for the great benefit of all people.

I want to strongly emphasize here that without receiving a reiki attunement it is not possible (or virtually 99.9999% impossible) to become a reiki practitioner. One must receive a reiki attunement from a live person who is in our direct presence, and who is in a direct line of transmission from O-Sensei. And yes, it is true that O-Sensei Usui received what is known as a "Universal Empowerment" or a "Divine Attunement" directly from the Universe (or God, Allah, the Buddha Realm, pick your words). But please note that he was also a highly unusually gifted and disciplined, and exquisitely and ultimately compassionate individual. O-Sensei Usui was "chosen" to open the path of reiki for all humanity, as a modern day Avatar of Healing and Compassion. The rest of us need to have a reiki attunement in the ordinary way - see a reiki teacher! It also cannot be received from a book, dvd, or website - despite the claims of many clever (or confused) marketers.

Now, I say this respectfully and compassionately. As a reiki sensei, however, I must be honest as well. We must not mislead ourselves or allow others to mislead us. And I say this also from a place of unique experience and training, having learned from many quite advanced and unusual lineage Grandmasters and Spiritual Teachers - some similar in league to O-Sensei himself. So humbly I only offer what they have taught me, and that my experience has proven to me - not mere personal opinion. Keep in mind, as well, that reiki is a perfect and fantastic teacher, for She is none other than our own Higher Self or Soul. I speak with Her daily and strive to follow Her lead and inspirations always. She is my muse, my Inner Guide, and my beloved best friend. This may sound strange, but She Herself has told me this - reiki attunement must be received from a live reiki teacher - there is no other proper way to become "reiki-fied".

So get thee to a good reiki teacher and have your "reiki light bulb" turned on, and your "reiki channel" tuned in! You won't regret it.

The Place of the Ego in Reiki

Quite simply, there is no place for the ego within the art of Usui Reiki Ryoho. It must be jettisoned completely from our consciousness, one way or another. The words of the Grandmaster Dr. Maung Gyi still ring in my ears, "There is absolutely no place for the ego in the context of reiki healing!" He also likes to put it this way: all thoughts of I, Me, Mine need to be eliminated.

This is perfectly in line with how the compassionate art of reiki operates, as well as how O-Sensei Usui was gifted with and developed and taught the art. As reiki practitioners we dedicate all to the Highest Good, whatever that may be, Thy Will Be Done, not mine... and release all attachments to the results or outcomes of our efforts. Thus, Usui Reiki Ryoho is like a kind of Karma Yoga or Bhakti Yoga, where we as reiki practitioners strive to operate from a place of universal love and compassion in order to cleanse, heal, and empower all. This includes ourselves, of course.

This cannot be done if we are operating from a place of delusion, division, and judgment (i.e. the ego). Keep in mind that we are all beloved sons and daughters of the same Universal Life Force, and equally beloved in Her eyes. From the seemingly highest to the seemingly lowest of us we are all deserving of love and compassion, respect and dignity, justice and freedom. How can my hand be above and/or better than my foot? Or my index finger more important than my elbow? Everything and everyone is completely interconnected and interdependent. We must humble ourselves to the point that we can once again be a part of the natural order of life and of Nature and the Universe. The ego divides and separates - the Universal Life Force brings all together.

One of my favorite quotes from Mahatma Gandhi is:

"The seeker after Truth must be lower than the dust which people grind under their feet each day as they walk down the street."

This is the level of egolessness which we must aspire to- but how to do it? Some recommend destroying the ego - kill it. Others say we must transcend the ego - fly away and fly above, leaving it behind. Still others say that the ego must be compassionately educated and healed, so that it may learn its proper place and function. Sort of like the tires on the car do not belong on the front hood - this would only blind us while we drive.

For reiki people it starts with daily contemplation of the "Gokai," or Reiki Life Principles, and striving to live these principles each and every day in all aspects of our lives. We will discuss the Gokai ("Five Principles") in the next chapter. Also, we should take the time to prepare and cleanse ourselves, and dedicate all to the Highest Good, Thy Will Be Done, not mine (or similar words/intent) before we begin any reiki healing or meditation session. In my book "The Compassionate Touch of Reiki: Healing Concepts, Elements, Methods" I describe in depth how to do this.

Another method of loosening the ego's iron-like grip upon our consciousness is to undergo a "thought fast" or "ego fast." Try to go for a specific amount of time without any thoughts of I, ME, or MINE. Say for ten minutes to begin with. And good luck with that one!

The best way to learn how to transcend the ego - which is one of the ways to healing and empowerment - is to find and learn from a truly advanced teacher/guide, one who has been on this path for a good portion of their lives. These teachers, the real ones, do exist but are not always easy to find. They can be like the mythical Dragon - pulsing with life force, powerful - but invisible!

Hint: in your search to find the "real thing" you cannot rely on titles, book or dvd sales, money, or other outer signs of success. It is not this simple - the "clothes" do not make the "Reiki Master." There are many charlatans and "snake oil" salesmen out there - so let the reiki buyer beware. Remember: the great Master from Palestine was a humble carpenter... the beggar on the street may be none other than Lord Buddha himself - the Immortal Ones generally don't advertise.

They say that, "when the student is ready the teacher appears." This is so very true. If you really desire to find and learn from a true Saint or Sage it can be done. Meditate upon this noble goal, keep it in your heart, and keep your eyes and ears open. Learn to listen to the "whispers of the Universe."

It took me one year to find my first teacher, over thirty years ago now. I knew that finding the right teacher was crucial, so I bided my time, until through an amazing synchronicity the Universe led us together. My teacher actually shook my hand and said, "We'll be here," as if he had been waiting for me. Keep in mind that with this art it is not like horseshoes or hand grenades - missing the mark by a little may lead us miles astray. This is where the teacher, a truly experienced and gifted one, comes into play to help make sure we don't miss the mark.

At a certain point, if we are truly disciplined and sincere, the Universe Herself will become our teacher. The reiki will teach us directly. But do not discount or diminish the role an advanced teacher can play in setting us on the right path and helping us to avoid mistakes. This is the way it has always been done. The great ones in sports, such as Larry Bird or Tiger Woods, still had coaches. In every field and every art and discipline (including reiki), this is vital.

Nowadays there is much too much importance placed upon titles in this art, to the point where they are completely meaningless, and worse, they are misleading and often used as tools to control people and/or rip them off. A real teacher or sensei is humble! They must be so, so humble. When we get caught up in our titles, with fame, with money or power and all the other outer and inner "ego traps" which exist, we risk crossing over to the "dark side." And I am not kidding! The compassionate art of reiki must never be practiced as a form of "black magic," either intentionally or unintentionally (as happens when the ego is overly prominent). And this path - the path of the ego - only leads to one place: darkness, death, pain, and suffering. I know, for I have been there. So stay away! Make a sacred oath to become the true embodiment of reiki- Universal Love and Compassion; and as I like to say (oops! I said it again):

"Be Real, Be Reiki."

Let me share with you an example of how my wise teacher once taught me this lesson, long ago now:

First of all, the lesson of egolessness (without losing power and confidence) was taught to us in endless ways from day one. But this specific example was quite memorable. After a period of two years of intensive training, practice, and testing I had earned the title of "Shr Shyung" or "Elder Brother" otherwise known as an assistant instructor of t'ai chi ch'uan. Although this was only the most basic level of instructorship available, given my teacher's lineage, reputation, and skill, this was quite an achievement. Very few students even made it to this basic level (it had nothing to do with money). Essentially this was compared to being a professor's assistant at an Ivy League school, in my mind anyway.

Keep in mind that I had begun training in great earnest, as for all intents and purposes my life had gone for a nose-dive off of the steep, rocky, cliffs of life: I had no parents, high blood pressure, depression, arthritis, poverty, abuse, and was "lost in space" when I found my teacher. The arts and concepts I was learning resonated from deep within me and were very healing and transformative. Because they basically had saved my life, I was extremely dedicated to my arts, my school, and my teacher. They were my oasis, my joy, my family, and my path.

So, like I say, achieving this first milestone - and I had big plans from day one, as all of us Capricorns do - as far as I was concerned was like being knighted by the King of England!

After successfully passing the tests, a day was appointed to hold a private ceremony to bestow the certificates upon the new or successful instructors and Sifu's who had taken the tests (testing was held four times a year, for those who were ready). This ceremony included the Headmaster, his close disciples, all the way down to us "newbies."

I'm kneeling there and the time comes for me to receive my diploma. Now, my teacher can have a very "heavy" presence and energy when he wants to. Well, he knows how focused (almost over focused) I had been to get to this point, and how important it was to me. So it's my turn and he decides at this point to teach me a lesson. Of course he didn't let on he was going to do this. Essentially he took all the "fun" out of it for me. But what a great lesson it was.

He's standing there in front of us holding my diploma and then goes into a long talk about how the certificate means nothing; it is worthless, not even worth the paper it was printed upon. He continues on saying that all such certificates and diplomas are, in fact, dead. They represent the past, which is over. As the art is a living art, we must live and practice the art each and every day if we are to be true practitioners. Then, to my complete mortification, he holds my certificate between his two hands and brings it to his mouth - and makes like he is going to rip it in half with his hands and teeth! Complete with hissing sound effects. Well, much to my relief he didn't actually rip it up, and having made his point he gave me the certificate - lesson taught, lesson received.

General Principles and Concepts of Reiki

"The real voyage of discovery lies not in finding new landscapes, but in having new eyes."

-Proust

The "General Concepts and Principles of Reiki" are fundamental to all aspects and applications of this compassionate art. They are interwoven seamlessly into the very fabric of the art to the point that in actuality they are what the fabric of reiki as an art of healing is made from. They make the art "tick," as it were.

In the next chapter we will examine the "Gokai," or Five Principles, which are another set of important concepts and principles. The "Gokai" are more of a reiki philosophy of living or life code; whereas the "General Concepts and Principles of Reiki" are more like seed and root principles and concepts. Let's explore them now:

1. Everything is Energy

The first important reiki general concept is that we are "spiritual/energetic beings having physical experiences" - not the other way around. Energy to us is as water is to a fish - we are so thoroughly dependent upon it and inundated by it that we take it for granted to the point of forgetting about it. Many people, even in this so-called "modern age," deny that life-force, or ch'i/ki/prana even exist. They believe that this is a fantasy which only the foolish, or children, believe in.

However, sticking to this outmoded and disproven belief is akin to believing that the Earth is flat and that the Sun revolves around this flat Earth, and the stars have been painted upon the sky by the Gods - literally.

I'm sorry to say, but the "joke" is on them. The truth is and has been proven many times over decades ago now (ever heard of $E=mc^2$?), that EVERYTHING is energy! There is actually very little - a completely tiny and miniscule amount - of matter which exists in the "materialized Universe." I read somewhere recently that in the span of one second a single atom will undergo trillions of energetic transformations. Trillions! So what does that compute out to be for a human being, or say, for planet Earth - untold trillions upon trillions upon trillions.

So we human beings are a part of an incomprehensibly huge, living energetic "being" which we call the Universe or the Cosmos. There is no denying it or getting around it. And this super energetic being is composed of probably unknowable amounts and varieties of energies. Some of which we are familiar with, such as gravity, radio waves, x-rays, and sunlight - but so many, many more we know nothing of, or are just beginning to learn about.

I am often bemused and befuddled when people express the view that something so obvious is actually not true, or even worse, they think something is "wrong" with you for speaking the obvious. Everything is energy, in a never ending process of evolving, maintaining, or transforming. Have you ever felt the sun on your skin? This is energy. Have you not seen the miracle of spring? Energy! Have you ever had a cut or would which healed? Again, energy. The examples which daily life provides for us exist in every moment for us to see if we would only open our eyes to see them. They are as close as our breath and our heartbeat - and in the toilet!

It is quite strange, as if some sort of black magic mind control spell has been cast over "modern man," that we will accept all manner of mechanical forms of energy. But mention natural, universal life-force-and this is thought to be so exotic or a delusion. My friends, you are alive! Thus, you have "life-force!" Do not be a stranger in your own body or your life or your world. An MRI, microwave ovens, the radio, tv, computers, pacemakers, cellphones - who among us questions their effectiveness? Yet they are dependent upon energy, are they not? The cell phone is my favorite example of our blindness and how we take energy for granted. As a child I grew up loving (a bit fanatically, I must admit) the classic American TV show from the 1960's Star Trek. Yes folks, I am indeed a sci-fi and fantasy nerd from way back. Well, occasionally my Mom - a fantastic, imaginative, and open-minded artist, but from an older generation - would glance at it as I watched Captain Kirk and crew and scratch her head. She didn't get it. I used to tell her that one day we would all have communicators like Captain Kirk - which for all intents and purposes is a cell phone. Her response? Yes you guessed it, a loving but firm, "No way, you're crazy!"

So everything is energy, everything is dependent on energy, and everything utilizes energy. Reiki is so very hard for many people to accept because it is such a pure and compassionate art of healing. I have even had people watching me give others reiki, in public demonstrations and workshops, actually heckle me. "You're not doing anything there" or "What do you think you are doing?" or better,

CHAPTER ONE: Essential Reiki Foundations

"You are just hypnotizing people." But hmm, I haven't moved or said anything. And much worse things than this they have said.

At my very first public lecture and demonstration of this art, at a large bookstore near me, I actually had a rather close-minded and stodgy fellow get up and stand between my audience and me and begin proclaiming that I was a dangerous cult leader! In a very excited way he exhorted the audience to be careful, or else crazy people like me would lead them to their death - look at Jim Jones and Jonestown! And he wasn't fooling around. Luckily no one bought or drank his "Kool-Aid."

How he made the leap from compassionate reiki healing to mass cult suicide I'll never know. Fear of the unknown combined with a traumatic past, perhaps. Needless to say, the demonstration ended early. As I walked away (yes, with steam coming out of my ears, I'm sorry to say), a very patient and compassionate member of the audience was trying to counsel and talk some sense to this guy. I heard him saying, "Brother, you need to open your mind," as I walked off.

When I told my very best friend (we were like true blood brothers) of reiki, he was convinced that I had joined a Satanic cult. The next time I visited him after telling him on the phone about reiki, he actually wouldn't let me into the house. He came out to the driveway to talk, as his family peered out of the windows at me like I was some sort of escaped and dangerous mental patient. He, and they, did get over this. They let me back in the house. With him it was childhood abuse he suffered at the hands of the Catholic Church which caused him to be so close-minded and confused about reiki.

I mention these episodes not to scare any potential reiki practitioners out there, but just to illustrate the level and depth of denial, confusion, and misinformation that there is out there. I would imagine other reiki people have similar stories to tell. Reiki, you see, just like viruses and bacteria, is invisible to the naked eye. And just like they are invisible yet real, so is reiki, but in a very positive way. When bacteria and viruses were discovered after the invention of the microscope and their role in disease was understood, it still took many decades for even hospitals and doctors to practice proper safety precautions, much less for the general public to understand. So at some point reiki and the concept that "Everything is Energy" will be accepted as common knowledge. We just aren't quite there yet.

Let me say again: reiki is the touch of the pure love and compassion of the Universe. This is a literal statement. Why are we so afraid of this? When you find the answer to this question you will have taken a giant step forward on the reiki path.

The reiki general concept – Everything Is Energy – symbolizes the Body of the Art of Reiki.

2. All Is One, We Are One

"Our task must be to free ourselves by widening our circle of compassion to embrace all beings and all of nature."

-Albert Einstein

The principle and concept of Unity, that All Is One, We Are One, is at the very core of what the energy of reiki and the art of Usui Reiki Ryoho is all about. It is the heart of the art, so to speak. Reiki is the fire of life which exists beyond all space and time. And simultaneously, reiki is the living web of light which connects all space, time, and dimensions together. Reiki is the union of the microcosm and the macrocosm, as well as their mother and father. She is truly a divine mystery.

When we receive reiki attunement the pathway to this timeless and unified dimension and state of consciousness is opened (permanently) so that healing of the total being may begin at an accelerated pace. Each one of us has our God and Higher Self appointed path and destiny or karma. Reiki and reiki attunement in no way interfere with this, they do not change us into someone or "something" else. It is not like "Invasion of the Reiki Body Snatchers"- quite the opposite of this, actually. As stated, what happens is that as individuals the pace and quality and the scope of healing can be supercharged. Like giving a plant the ideal conditions with which to grow, along with perfect nutrients. As I have described, reiki acts like a spiritual/energetic cleanser, tonic, and transformational energy upon us. It helps us to be the best that we can be given the circumstances we may find ourselves in, following the concept of "flower and bloom where you are planted." Exactly how this manifests is potentially unlimited. For instance, reiki is highly beneficial for hospice patients. However, by receiving reiki healing and attunement we should not assume that they are going to be miraculously "cured" and get up and go home, for everything born at some point passes on. This is a natural part of the Circle of Life. The Universal Life Force is never static, She is always transforming one way or another.

However, the hospice patients may find that the reiki helps them to experience greater peace, less pain, and to find a way to gracefully accept the situation. This of course in turn positively impacts all around them: their family, friends, and even the hospice staff working with them. So reiki provides healing and a great blessing for all involved.

CHAPTER ONE: Essential Reiki Foundations

So, we are who we are, but at the same time, all things change. Ahh, I can't help it, for that old piece of well-known wisdom has just popped into my head: "The only thing that doesn't change is change itself."

Now I must be very sensitive with my next comments, as I mean no disrespect to anyone or to any group, and I am certainly not here to tell anyone what to think or how to live. However, humbly I offer these ideas for people to honestly and sincerely contemplate, as they are key to understanding reiki and reiki healing properly:

Reiki attunement greatly opens our inner pathways to healing and connects us very powerfully to the unlimited, eternal, pure and perfect "Higher Realm." The names for this pure and perfect realm are legion: Heaven, Buddha's Pure Realm, the Sach Khand, and many others. So naturally, as a consequence of this, reiki attunement and reiki healing will work to heal our consciousness. This great art is no mere energetic healing art with which we patch up our little (or giant) blown out and cut up energetic tires with! As we have stated - and has been taught by O-Sensei and proven by his example and by the lives of untold reiki people - reiki and the art of reiki are indeed a true life path and Dao of living. As we travel this path and experience the great gifts of inner healing, naturally our consciousness begins to heal. We may begin to find that we are becoming truly happy and peaceful, from inside our hearts and our minds. We may become more relaxed, and feel a great connection within and to all around us, including other people - even the difficult and challenging ones. After all, who hasn't had a bad day?

This hit me very soon after receiving my first reiki attunement. I can be a naturally driven person, always out to prove myself and be the best. Yes, I am a Capricorn's Capricorn, I used to practically plan each and every step I took and move I made. Alright, I still do, but with the help and counseling of reiki I am much more relaxed about it and schedule "down time." As I have mentioned and described a bit, I have had a stressful life, to stay the least. Well, after my first reiki class I began giving myself reiki every day. One morning a while after this in early spring, I awoke around dawn very peacefully and just laid there. As I lay there I listened to the great blessing and the miracle of the birds singing and welcoming the new spring sun at dawn. And as I lay there and the birds sang, it hit me that it had been many, many years since I had slowed down enough and been relaxed and open enough to experience this simple pleasure and gift which Nature provides for us each and every day. What a blessing and great healing this was for me. My teacher's words of wisdom became very clear to me at this time, as well, "the farther mankind gets from nature, the more neurotic he becomes."

So, We Are One, All Is One. As our consciousness is healed within and we come to recognize this as being the truth, so many artificial barriers and cruel, false human constructions may come crashing down or fade away.

One of my students told me that growing up she experienced so much pain and suffering due to a teaching that had been ingrained into her head from early childhood by her church. They told her that everyone who did not follow their beliefs was going to Hell, a most unpleasant fate. And they were quite vivid and detailed in describing the eternal suffering and damnation they would be condemned to in this infernal place. Being by nature so very intuitive and compassionate, she cried and cried over this. This meant that many of the people she loved - her friends at school, friends from the neighborhood, her teachers, and all good people whom she loved dearly of different belief systems - were going to be tortured eternally in Hell, according to what the authorities in her life were telling her. And being such a compassionate and sensitive child, it broke her heart and wounded her deeply.

As she grew older she began to think about this more logically. You mean, Mother Teresa and Mahatma Gandhi and the Reverend Dr. Martin Luther King, Jr. are all going to Hell as well, despite being such ultimately compassionate and saintly human beings? Hmmm, she thought and thought about this, and eventually after undergoing much inner healing was able to move past and let go of this false teaching. And after some more time and more healing she was even able to forgive the ones who had first implanted this horrible and wicked concept and false teaching into her young and sensitive mind. This was indeed a great healing for her, one which reiki helped to facilitate.

Years ago I was able to meet and receive teachings and initiation/shaktipat directly from a famous and true living saint, H. H. Sant Rajinder Singh Ji Maharaj. He is one of the world's great interfaith spiritual leaders. Well, the entire day - and the time since I met him - was and has been profoundly eventful. His energy and the words of wisdom he shared with us I can never forget. At one point during his opening satsang he talked about some things that are directly relevant regarding the Unity of All. In fact, it was the major theme of his divine discourse. He explained quite logically that when the great Teachers, Saints, Sages, and Prophets come that they do not discriminate.

To paraphrase, he said it this way: "Jesus did not come just for Christians. There were no Christians in his time! Jesus came for all people!" Continuing on in the same vein, he emphasized again, "Buddha did not come just for the Buddhists - for there were no Buddhists at first. Buddha came for all people!" And he continued on like this, mentioning several other of the great religious

CHAPTER ONE: Essential Reiki Foundations

and spiritual leaders of world history. There was so much truth in his words, they touched me very deeply. To put it in terms reiki people will appreciate, we are all children of the same Universal Life Force, and equally beloved in Her eyes. And also, though there may be many paths up the mountain - there is only One Mountain we all must climb.

The great Guru Nanak (The Prophet of the Sikh religion) was beloved by all the people of his time. His students included both Hindus and Muslims; which if you know anything about the explosive history between these groups, is quite unusual. His teachings reflect the wisdom of both paths as well, in a beautiful fusion illustrating again that truly, All is One.

So, as we have learned now, reiki is the pure energy of the Grace, and the Love and the Compassion of the Universal Life Force and of the Source. She is above and beyond all concepts of division and judgment, which we humans may artificially construct. In the Christian Holy Bible there is a famous statement and teaching, "God said, 'Let there be light,' and there was light." This sound and this light is none other than the reiki Herself. She existed before (as well as above and beyond) any human dogma was created. This teaching is fundamental to many religions, spiritual paths, and mystic revelations all over the world. And it connects us all together. When we discuss "Reiki Unity Healing" - otherwise known as "distance healing" (enkaku chiryo-ho) - later in this book, we will delve into this topic even more. And as reiki practitioners we can all learn to live in this high state of blissful consciousness as well; one reflecting pure Love and Unity, as we are meant to live.

The age of "an eye for an eye, and a tooth for a tooth" and of "you are either with us or you are against us" is over. Their usefulness, if there was ever any, is long gone now. They are dangerous relics of a bygone era. Reiki is not a religion, it is a path which all of us may follow and equally benefit from. Thus, She is a perfect art and teaching for this modern and interdependent age we find ourselves in, one in which discord anywhere directly affects us all. As we can now, as equal sons and daughters of the same Universal Life Force, we should all try to embrace this great concept and teaching, and let the artificial barriers fall down and fade away: All Is One, We Are One.

This reiki concept symbolizes the Mind of the art of reiki.

3. Spirit (reiki) Commands Energy

This important principle is the one which is responsible for the complete ease, naturalness, and safety of the art of Usui Reiki Ryoho, as well as for its potential power and effectiveness. As we have discussed, reiki is none other than an aspect of the Divine Source. The words for these concepts may vary, but as the Great Bard so eloquently put it long ago, "A rose by any other name would still smell as sweet." So let's not get hung up on terms.

This is a well-known internal arts teaching - <u>Spirit (reiki) Commands Energy</u>. In the context of the art of Usui Reiki Ryoho, what this means is that in all applications and aspects of reiki healing and reiki attunement, the purity and power of the energy of reiki is potentially able to bring balance and harmony, as well as vitality and vibrancy, to the total being. Again, the energy of reiki may act as a cleansing and purifying agent, as a tonic and vitalizing power, and/or as an energy which brings balance and harmony.

A human being (or any living being) will absorb and make use of the reiki in a process which is similar to digestion. Since the energy, as an aspect of the Source, is so pure and potent, the human energy system has virtually no block to receiving and making positive use of it. Reiki is completely essential, fundamental, and in tune with all other energies which a human being may make use of. Quite simply, it is the Source energy of all. Thus, it is transformed into, and is utilized by, all other energies and energetic processes that a human being needs and makes use of - energies of spirit, mind, and body. Reiki, thereby, helps to bring balance, order, and harmony to the total being - by "commanding" all other energies and energetic processes.

Now, this is a huge and complex topic which deserves its own book to do it justice - the total process of how reiki spiritual energy work and healing/attunement technically works. Here I am interested in only introducing the basics so that people will have a general understanding of this topic. The good news is that because the compassionate art of reiki is almost completely a non-technical and natural one, even children or illiterate people can safely - and with great results - make use of the art. Like breathing and our heartbeat, sunrise and sunset, reiki is natural and happens whatever our knowledge of these things may be.

I would refer interested people again to Dr. Daniel Reid's most wonderful book, "A Complete Guide to the Principles and Practices of Chi-Gung" (Shambhala Publications) for an in-depth discussion and presentation of this topic. In reading this, or similar works, on human spiritual/energy systems, the chakras, the dantien system, core channels, meridians, and the like (there are thousands of energetic systems, by the way) keep in mind that Usui Reiki Ryoho is very unique. How the process of spiritual/energetic healing operates and is conducted with this art is different than in virtually all other arts, in various ways. This is due, primarily, to the marvelous qualities of the reiki energy Herself, and the great gift of reiki attunement. Both of which are gifts from the

CHAPTER ONE: Essential Reiki Foundations

Universe, and shared with all humanity now due to the great achievement and ultimate compassion of the Founder, O-Sensei Usui.

It's important to practice reiki as I am explaining it and not to mix systems, as it takes an extremely experienced and intuitive reiki teacher or practitioner to properly translate the concepts and practices of one art to this one (and vice-versa). For instance, the principles and rules of classical piano are quite different than those of heavy, acid-rock guitar playing, Jimi Hendrix style. Even though they are both forms of music, it would take an expert virtuoso to blend them properly. I would love to hear this, by the way! So don't jump to conclusions and think all of these "energy arts" are the same, so they may be easily mixed and matched like Lego-blocks. Uh-uh, sorry. As my martial arts teacher taught me early on, "a little bit of knowledge is dangerous."

What is most important for reiki people to learn is how to practice the art simply and safely, and then to be disciplined about practicing and living it.

The theories and concepts underlying the art are quite secondary, so don't get too hung up on them. Reiki is a completely natural art, this should never be forgotten. The key to being a reiki person is to utilize the art regularly, and to live the art and Her principles of compassion in daily life. Just as studying art history will not make one into an artist, studying reiki theory may or may not be helpful. Don't forget: "Be Real, Be Reiki."

In terms a practitioner of Chinese Chi-Gung (qigong) would understand, Usui Reiki Ryoho could be called "Usui's Living Ch'i Gung Dao." To a yogic arts practitioner, the art of reiki is way beyond ordinary "pranic healing." She is a unique and powerful transformative spiritual art making use of none other than the divine "maha para shakti." And I mean no disrespect to practitioners of other, similar arts. They all, of course, have their strengths.

Each and every spiritual/energy healing art is unique - and Usui Reiki Ryoho is no exception. They can't and shouldn't all be lumped together into one generic "Energy Healing" category, as if they are all the same. This is much too simplistic. The little toy cars children play with are all cars of a sort, but can they be compared to a real Mercedes or Jaguar? I don't think so. In just the same way, this great art should not be equated with other arts. They may share very little in common, other than some minor outward appearances.

We must remember that O-Sensei Usui was not just a highly knowledgeable and experienced teacher and scholar. He was also a real Saint and Avatar who underwent a powerful and life altering enlightenment experience while fasting atop sacred Mt. Kurama. He was a spiritual giant whom all who met and got to know him were in awe of. O-Sensei received a "Divine Attunement," a "Universal Empowerment" akin to a gift which keeps on giving. A gift which lives on, via reiki attunement, in each and every reiki student who is alive, has lived, or will ever live. The truth is that O-Sensei should rightly be thought of as an Avatar of Compassion and Healing. Avatars are beings which rarely visit the Earth, they come in times of great need and are able to fundamentally change the nature of human society and human consciousness; in one way or another and to one level or another. It is interesting to note that O-Sensei himself described this as exactly being his mission, and what his art was for (see the Reiki Ryoho Hikkei). And of course this is happening, witness the untold millions upon millions of reiki people all over the Earth now, and the acceptance of the art now - all of which serves to elevate human consciousness and bring us together. I mention all of this as an example of this principle - <u>Spirit (reiki) Commands Energy</u> - at the macrocosmic, world level. Reiki operates in all levels and dimensions, always for the highest good of all (our next principle).

So have no fear, we reiki people are not some kind of demonic, invisible, terrorist sleeper-cell cult. Quite the contrary: we are all members of the United Forces of Love, Light, and Compassion- with love for all, and all for love.

This reiki concept – Spirit (reiki) Commands Energy – symbolizes the Heart of the art of reiki.

"In this modern era human happiness is based on living and working together and a desire for social development... Our method is something completely original, there is nothing like it in the whole world Therefore, I want to share it with the public for the benefit of all humanity."

-O-Sensei Mikao Usui, from the Reiki Ryoho Hikkei

---

4. Thy Will Be Done, not mine

This reiki principle is the one which symbolizes the intent of all possible applications of the art of Usui Reiki Ryoho. It also allows for the higher level healing aspects of the art to manifest - the spiritual healing aspects - and differentiates it from simple, low-level "energy healing" arts which generally address symptoms only. The compassionate touch of reiki, of course, can and does aid in relieving symptoms of imbalance: stress, pain, anxiety, and the like, but she also works directly from the core outwards and may be followed as a Life Path, as we have discussed and as O-Sensei conceived of and transmitted his art.

Another way of saying this - Thy Will Be Done, not mine - is that as reiki practitioners we must strive to extinguish the small self and live from the Higher Self. And we must acknowledge this and dedicate all applications of reiki to this.

Truly, as we shall explore in more detail later in this book and in the second volume of this series, there are no limits to the application of reiki healing. Reiki is the Universal Life Force, thus Her applications are indeed universal and not even limited by space or time. Keep in mind that All Is One. We start, generally, with the simple and mundane - basic hands on reiki healing methods for self and others along with simple reiki meditations. This is in order to gain experience and to be healthy and balanced in spirit, mind, and body. After that the sky is the limit- and go for it, aim for the stars, who knows, you might become one. After all, we are all already bright, shining stars in the soul ... most of us have just forgotten. The compassionate touch of reiki helps us to remember this beautiful truth.

Another healing maxim which I love and which works well with this one is the old Wiccan injunction, "an' it harm none, do as ye will." After all, at least in theory and in soul, as Higher Self, we are all free beings and deserving to be able to live our lives as we see fit - with respect to all and for all, and dedicating all to the Highest Good. After this, live how you like to, dress how you like to, talk to whom you want to, believe what you will believe, love who you love - we each have our own journey to lead and path to follow as we climb the mountain of Life. And we should all be free to follow our own path, "if it harm none."

Each of these principles and concepts - along with the Gokai - all interact with and balance each other. Until we connect with our own source of inner wisdom it can be a bit confusing, so do your best. Always err on the side of kindness, compassion, respect, and freedom, if you are unsure.

I would like to note here that the opposite of this principle (Thy Will Be Done, not mine) is to simply "Do as ye will" or "My Will Be Done, I Will Do What I Want." Why do I mention this? Any philosophy, teaching, organization, individual, "religion, " church, temple, or cult which has integrated and promotes this teaching - "Do What You Want" is actually propagating Satanic principles, or what is otherwise known as "black magic."

Now I know some of you reading this are thinking, "wow, this guy is superstitious!" But it all comes down to energy. Are we practicing and promoting teachings and energy which contribute to the greater good, to freedom, and to the positive evolution of all; or ones which promote chaos, slavery, and destruction?

In other words, are we emissaries of the Light or of the Shadow? And we all have free will, so choose wisely young Jedi. The Star Wars movies vividly portray the consequences of these choices, and the redemptive healing power of forgiveness. Thanks be to Mr. George Lucas and all involved for bringing them to the world. Wisdom and Light may be found everywhere so keep yourself open to them. Even at the movies...

This is a very sensitive and complex topic. For now keep in mind that as High and Mighty and Glorious as the Light is in this Universe - just this high, but in a diabolic way, is the Shadow. And the Shadow can be very deceiving. He may appear in the most appealing of forms. So choose your path wisely, listen to your heart.

This reiki principle and concept – Thy Will Be Done, not mine – symbolizes the Way (Dao) of Reiki.

Summary of General Reiki Concepts and Principles:

1. <u>The Body of the Art</u> - "Everything is Energy"

2. <u>The Mind of the Art</u> - "All is One, We Are One"

3. <u>The Heart of the Art</u> - "Spirit (reiki) Commands Energy"

4. <u>The Way (Dao) of the Art</u> - "Thy Will Be Done, not mine"

What is the Butterfly Reiki System?

"Other men are clear and bright, but I alone am dim and weak. Other men are sharp and clever, but I alone am dull and stupid."

-Lao Tzu[4]

As I mentioned in the preface, B.R.S. is quite simply my own unique presentation of Usui Reiki Ryoho. Thus, B.R.S. is a modem manifestation of Usui Reiki Ryoho, plain and simple. It is not some newly discovered "ancient secret" nor is it the freshly revealed teachings of the divine Immortal Sages which were "whispered into my ears" during a trance-state, or anything like that. I am not attempting to reinvent the wheel - or even sliced bread! It's already been done.

It would be silly and preposterous of me (though my ego might like it) to think that I could improve upon the marvelous and perfect teachings of a Sage and Saint such as O-Sensei Usui. Or even of his disciples, many of which were quite remarkable and powerful people in their own right, as well as being highly advanced reiki and spiritual teachers.

Before I describe technically what the B.R.S. is as a reiki system, let me share with you my "reiki story" as it is useful as an example of the healing power of this compassionate art, and will give you a better idea of where I am coming from formulating the B.R.S.

How Reiki Found Me:

I first heard of reiki when I ran across a book in a bookstore. It was intriguing, but presented the art in an extremely "New Age-y" manner, rather than as an Asian art of healing. And let me say that I was beyond skeptical after seeing this book - I was openly and vociferously derisive of this great art. I have since learned to temper my initial opinions of such things, as there is always more to learn. But you see, based upon my previous years of experience and intense training - as a student, practitioner, instructor, Sifu, and Lineage Disciple in

---

[4] Excerpt from *Tao TeChing,* Chapter 20, Gia Fu Fong and Jane English translation.

arts as diverse as t'ai chi ch'uan (taijiquan), ch'i gung (qigong) and nei gung (nei gong), meditation styles of all kinds, Five Formed Fist Shaolin Ch'uan-fu, Filipino martial arts, various yoga styles and methods, and any and all other related martial, meditative, healing, and metaphysical arts which I found interesting and valuable - I fancied myself an "expert." This was in the mid 1990's. When I read in this book that anyone could receive the gift of reiki healing ability easily, simply, and effortlessly, honestly I thought that the author (in her biography picture she wore flowing white robes) was simply taking advantage of poor, witless, idealistic but ignorant, mush-brained "New Agers!" You must understand that unfortunately, there is a huge market out there for this. There are so many, many schemes and scams for ripping off ignorant and/or confused and idealistic people-this includes in the so-called "spiritual/religious" fields and all others. This is not cynical talk, either. It just happens to be a sad fact. What is that old piece of wisdom? "A fool and his money are easily parted." As a recent and (in)famous U.S. President said, taking P.T. Barnum's observation one step farther, "you can fool some of the people all of the time - and those are the ones you want to concentrate on."

Have you heard the joke about the politician, the religious leader, the gangster and the prostitute? It goes like this: what is the difference between them? Answer: there is none, they just wear different clothes.

Anyway, so I thought that the great and compassionate art of reiki was worse than a bad joke - it might be nothing more than a scheme to rip people off! However, it did stick in my mind, and as I try to balance having a discerning mind with having an open one, and loving to learn new things; eventually I was led to giving this seemingly silly, exotic, and strange art a shot. I had just moved to a new area of the state of Connecticut, and near me a small local hospital was having a free "Integrative Healing Arts Day." This included demonstrations of the various arts the hospital was offering to the public, as well as free food and music - and reiki healing sessions. So I figured, this is the perfect chance to find out about this weird reiki stuff, and if nothing else I'll meet some new people and have a nice meal (see how sneaky I can be?).

Well, even as I was pulling into the parking lot I began sensing one of those feelings you get that life and fate are about to tap you on the shoulder - or perhaps smack you upside the head. I walked in thinking to myself, "hmm, something seems to be going on here that is for real but...?" and beheld a lovely scene: fresh, healthy foods, nice, smiling people, a live flute player, t'ai chi and yoga demonstrations, and the like. After taking it in for a minute, I walked over to the table where they were signing people up for thirty-minute reiki sessions, and sat down to sign up. As I did so I struck up a conversation

CHAPTER ONE: Essential Reiki Foundations

with the young lady doing the sign-up; a beautiful, blue-eyed blonde of twenty, later I found out that her mom was one of the people sharing the free reiki sessions with the public.

Now, I was sitting in a long and wide hallway, the table was in front of me, the beautiful young lady was to my left, and the large conference room/reiki room was to my right. Since reiki people had been in there reiki-ing away for hours, I am describing this scene to you because it became my first introduction to the power of reiki - and a most amazing one.

I was about twenty-eight years old at the time, and this young lady had my full attention. The reason for my visit was no longer my immediate priority, you could say. As we spoke and began to develop a rapport, all of a sudden the right side of my body - the side facing the reiki healing room - began getting deliciously and pleasantly warm and tingly! And I mean from head to toe, the whole right side of my body - and this room was about fifteen feet away. So I mentioned this to my new friend and she smiled and sweetly said, "why do you think I am sitting here?"

Please note, for the skeptical readers out there, this was in no way some sort of self-implanted autosuggestion or self-hypnosis on my part. As I have described, I was definitely not thinking about the reiki or the reiki healing room. As the female readers know - and us tortured males may have experienced - there are few powers on Earth which can overcome the power a beautiful woman can have over us hapless and helpless males, especially at that age. Well, guess what? Reiki is one of those powers! But this was only the beginning to an amazing day...

So after enjoying the conversation and wonderful new sensations I was experiencing, it was my turn for an "official" reiki session. As I lay on the reiki table I received one of the most remarkable experiences of my life - I phased in and out of consciousness, as if drifting from dream to dream. My body went completely limp, like warm jello. Delicious, warm, tingly sensations coursed through my body. And thirty minutes passed by in an instant. When my magical new reiki friend was done, she helped me off the table, as I was literally left dazed and speechless by the experience. I was barely able to walk to the corner of the room, whereupon I had to sit down on the floor for an hour to let it all integrate and pass - the reiki session had been so powerful and had relieved such stress and touched me so deeply that I literally couldn't stand, much less drive home. So after an hour of sitting, breathing, and taking it all in, I was able to float off and find my car.

On the ride home I was able to summon the strength, out of nowhere (remember I went into this experience as a skeptic) to quit drinking coffee, immediately and on the spot. At the time I was drinking ten to twenty cups of black coffee a day. I didn't need even one cup, as naturally I have energy like the Energizer Bunny. The coffee was just filling an emotional need - and causing me to bounce of walls! So like I say, I drove away and swore to myself that I would quit, and I did. For four years after that I didn't have one cup of coffee, enjoying green tea and other herbal teas as a much healthier beverage. And even more unbelievable, I had no caffeine withdrawal symptoms when I quit.

Obviously I was beyond intrigued by all of this, and by this awesome new art at this point- I wanted to learn immediately, which I did, getting in touch initially with the people I had met at the hospital. It's been a wonderful, strange but beautiful, enlightening, and at times even frightening journey since then.

So this was my initial introduction to the compassion and power of reiki, and She made quite an impression on me. The B.R.S., however, has been developed from the sum-total of my life experiences. And oftentimes, unfortunately, from birth these were the opposite of what I saw on TV with shows like Leave it to Beaver or The Brady Bunch. But it was these experiences that led me to the path which led me to Her, so I give thanks for them and their lessons.

Poverty, abuse - sexual, physical, verbal, emotional, hunger, loss and abandonment, pain and suffering - I have experienced them all, since entering this world. To the point that by the time I was twenty years old I had no parents (my Mom had died horribly from cancer, and good ole Pops was a distant and painful memory), high blood pressure of 165 over 110, depression, and arthritis. I mention these things not to complain or to look for sympathy, but rather to illustrate the awesome and compassionate power of reiki and related inner meditative healing arts, of which reiki is the Queen.

As I sit here and write I find myself happy, healthy, and at peace. Both with myself and with my world, more so than I can remember for many, long years. Happiness and peace truly come from within, and reiki has led me to find this sacred blessing within myself.

Back to my reiki "story." It was at this point, as a semi-broken but not beaten twenty year old (after my Mom had passed) that I vowed to take charge of my sinking ship and to change my life. From birth I had been interested in martial arts, having grown up watching and being fascinated by the exploits of the incomparable Bruce Lee and the wise Kwai Chang Caine of Kung Fu fame. As we were dirt poor - I wore my friends' clothes and my mom cut my hair - I began to study from books around the age of eight. In fact, I still have my first two martial arts books, excellent books with many photos, geared for children - one on judo and one on karate. How my mom was able to scrape the money together to buy these for me I do not know, but out of her great love for me she did. So I studied and practiced what I saw in those books - they both had a graduated study program that went up to "black belt" - much to the chagrin of my practice partner, my younger sister. At a certain point I even arranged for my mom to give me a formal "belt test." And yes, thanks to mom, I earned my first two black belts! Thanks, Mom.

Anyway, like I say, by age twenty I was a mess and needed to bring order to my chaotic and painful young life. So I decided to begin formal training in martial arts, and over the course of one year I researched and looked for just the right art for me (as I needed healing, not just fighting), and most importantly, the right school and teacher. You see, I was quite determined about this resolution, and wanted to get it right from the start and waste no time. As the old saying goes, "when the student is ready, the teacher appears." Seemingly by chance, as I was not having any luck finding a proper t'ai chi instructor- most of the ones I did find at this point (around 1986) seemed to know less than I did, and I hadn't even formally trained yet. Plus I was looking for "for real" traditional t'ai chi, not the "New Age" version; the modern "sport" t'ai chi version didn't even really exist yet here in the U.S. at that time; but has since, unfortunately, taken over. No interest in that, either.

Well, as I say, one day as I was driving my sister's friend home I literally almost crashed my car into my teacher's school, while on the passenger seat next to me was a letter I just received recommending his school to me. Can you say "synchronicity?" "Karma?" Call it what you want, but to make a long story short, due to my teacher's great knowledge, skills, abilities, and programs - as well as those of the many other great teachers, healers, and spiritual teachers and leaders I have been blessed to meet and learn from (combined with my own stubbornness and discipline) - here I am!

On my journey to developing the Butterfly Reiki System I have been so extremely fortunate to have been able to learn from and be blessed by - through initiation, empowerment, darshan, satsang, and shaktipat - a variety of teachers, Saints, and Sages of diverse lineages, some of which who are in the same league as O-Sensei Usui himself. For what these people have done for me I have no words which can adequately thank them.

When I began my healing journey I was almost lost without a trace, on a nose-dive off of the steep and rocky cliffs of life. There is not nor will there ever be enough money, gold, and treasure to repay them. To carry on what they have shared with me, faithfully and in as true a fashion as I can, is my gift in return. As it has always been, the Circle of Life is Eternal: life to life, person to person, generation to generation. Until the work is completed and all have been enlightened. Namaste.

What Makes a Butterfly?

Technically, the Butterfly Reiki System is composed of the seven main elements of the traditional Usui Reiki Ryoho. These are what I call the Seven Jewels of Reiki, and we will explore them in the next chapter and in much more depth especially in my book "The Compassionate Touch of Reiki: Healing Concepts, Elements, Methods" which also introduces the curriculum for the first two levels of the Butterfly Reiki System (Shoden and Chuden).

Keep in mind that with the B.R.S. I am not trying to faithfully recreate exactly what and how O-Sensei taught his art, as if unearthing and presenting to the public an archeological treasure or artifact. This is neither appropriate nor desirable. I am an American and as I write it is the year 2011. O-Sensei was a Japanese Saint and Avatar who passed on in 1926. We are different people, the world is different now, and the cultures we operate in are vastly different. As are the people I work with, as compared to those whom O-Sensei worked with. People are people, true.

But people of differing times and cultures can be so different in many ways that we may as well be aliens. Thus, presenting an art like reiki may vary a bit depending upon the time and place it is being shared. And this can easily be done without losing the essence of what the Founder intended his art to be. Arts like reiki which don't evolve and change with the time and place they are in become "dead arts" very quickly.

Thus, what I am attempting to do with the B.R.S. is to bring to life more of the traditional essence and intent of this great, compassionate art. As the Founder intended it to be. The essence of the art is nothing anyone can see or read about. It is beyond any of its techniques and methods, as well. One could faithfully memorize every technique and all of the known facts regarding O-Sensei and his art and still be light years from the essence, from the source. As Basho has so perfectly put it, "Seek not to follow in the footsteps of the Ancient Masters - seek what they sought!" Find this and you will have the essence of reiki.

So I am attempting to revive the tradition and essence of reiki. At the same time, I am also interested in improving and clarifying people's understanding of the art - what it is and isn't - as well as improving the actual technique and methods, which have become very weak and watered down.

For instance, reiki meditation and reiki-ko are vital elements of Usui Reiki Ryoho. Now, whether one practices exactly the same methods as O-Sensei and his disciples is secondary. What is primary is that reiki students practice reiki meditation and reiki-ko! The possibilities in actual technique are virtually limitless - but reiki people must "just do it." As I say, people in one culture and time may be drawn to various styles and methods, but this is only natural and as it should be. People also enjoy different styles and types of pizza all over planet Earth - but we all enjoy pizza, don't we? Mmm, pizza.

So the B.R.S. has been constructed from and modeled upon the traditional essence of Usui Reiki Ryoho, officially since 1997 - I didn't just dream her up yesterday. B.R.S. is composed primarily of universal concepts and methods which all people may learn, practice, and enjoy. Meaning I try to keep them as free of any specific religious-dogmatic overtones as possible.

Reiki is a gift for all of humanity, and unites all humanity. So ideally our "reiki dogma" should be as pure and universal as possible. Though of course, there are so many reiki styles now that there are indeed untold of what I call "reiki theme arts" - Buddhist Reiki, Christian Reiki, Egyptian Mystical Reiki, New Age Reiki, Tibetan Reiki, and much more- but I have purposely avoided this with the B.R.S. so that she will be, hopefully, of interest to the widest audience as possible.

Some of the methods and concepts utilized and taught in the B.R.S. are quite unique and unknown to the wider reiki world and come from my experiences learning from highly evolved and unusual teachers with ancient and authentic Asian lineages. Some of the methods and concepts are well known to the wider reiki world. And still others are partially known, such as the various traditional Japanese reiki methods.

Specifically, I have studied and learned reiki arts as diverse as Takata and Hayashi style reiki, Usui/Tibetan reiki, traditional Japanese reiki, Buddho/Enersense and Reiki Jin Kei Do, Essential Reiki, Karuna© reiki, and anything and everything else "reiki" that I could find information on. And of course my background in ch'i gung and nei gung; Min Zin and rare reiki methods; various meditation styles - from the well-known to the quite esoteric; t' ai chi, kung fu, and martial arts in general; and various other spiritual, energetic, and mystical arts, concepts, and methods are all appropriately blended into and factored into the Butterfly Reiki System. All this makes the B.R.S. one of the most unique, comprehensive, yet traditional and effective reiki methods out there - in my humble opinion, anyway.

Most importantly, I preserve and teach the traditional intent of how the art should be learned, practiced, and taught. Specifically this means that kindness and compassion must be balanced with humility and discipline; and openness and availability with discernment and reality (i.e. the Truth). Read and contemplate the Gokai and O-Sensei's actual words and you will see this is how we are meant to conceive of and live the art - in balance. In fact, it is said that O-Sensei's "Dojo Motto" was "Unity of Self through Harmony and Balance." This maxim perfectly describes the path and the goals of this compassionate art. Oh, and by the way, there isn't a payment plan for these things no matter how much "reiki" you buy on the internet. Sorry to say, but it is what it is.

In O-Sensei's day people learned and practiced reiki in a Reiki Dojo - like setting under the direct guidance of expert teachers. And more importantly, reiki students had to "carry the art into the field," or live the art in the true dojo of everyday life - the only real school we all have. The training was viewed as a life-long journey, a journey towards self-realization and enlightenment ("personal perfection" as O-Sensei called it). Compare this to the modern way in which reiki is often "taught," where someone just goes to a website and poof! Shazaam! They are instantly conferred, quote-unquote, "Reiki Master" status! Yay! Congratulations! But is it really this simple? Really? Reality check time: it is interesting to note that neither O-Sensei Usui nor any of his disciples - nor their disciples (such as Reverend Takata) - ever taught the art in such a commercialized and fast-food fashion. Ever!

Yes, it is possible that modern technology can assist in the learning process, no doubts about this. But as they say, "let the buyer beware." Reiki is indeed a simultaneously simple yet profound art available easily to all people, even children. This is absolutely true. It's just that properly learning, and especially "mastering the art" is not so simple. Think about it, if you went online and bought a "college diploma" for a couple of hundred dollars - would this actually be the same as earning one by attending and graduating with a Masters Degree from a legitimate and accredited college or university? If you believe so, perhaps you would like to buy this land I have for sale.

I remember once, years ago, a lady walked into my teacher's school and declared that she had "already mastered all of the laws of the universe." All she wanted from him was for him to teach her some techniques. My jaw dropped when I heard and saw this. Well, my so wise teacher told her that if this was indeed the case, then she didn't need him. And he dismissed her! What a great lesson this was for her. I hope she learned it, and ate some "humble pie." Whatever happened to "practice makes perfect?" There is so much more I could say here, but for now we will leave it at this and let the thoughtful reader contemplate the true path of reiki. Hint: it must be walked and walked

The Seven Jewels of Reiki

and walked, day in and day out- forever! Then maybe, just maybe, *if* you are blessed and extremely sincere and disciplined, you will be recognized as a "Master of Reiki." May good fortune smile upon you on your journey.

"If you master one circle, have you mastered all circles?"

-Zen Koan

Why Reiki?

"When the world is in possession of the Tao,
The galloping horses are led to fertilize the fields with their droppings.
When the world becomes Taoless,
War horses breed themselves on the suburbs.
There is no calamity like not knowing what is enough.
There is no evil like covetousness.
Only he who knows what is enough will always have enough."

- Lao Tzu[5]

In this first chapter we have discussed many of the important and essential elements and concepts of reiki and of Usui Reiki Ryoho. The compassionate art of reiki is truly ideal for all people. She safely, simply, and effectively promotes health and balance for spirit, mind, and body. These are blessings we all are in need of.

We live in very challenging times. There is an old Chinese "curse," perhaps you have heard it, "may you live in interesting times." Well, my friends, we certainly are, aren't we? And no doubt for the foreseeable future they may indeed become even more "interesting." As a compassionate art of healing, reiki promotes many positive qualities, as I have already described and we will see in great depth and detail in the rest of this book. Chief among these qualities are achieving and maintaining balance and harmony. But what does this mean?

Quite simply this means avoiding extremes and living and being in tune with the flow of life and Nature - the Universal Life Force. We are all living expressions of the same Universal Life Force, we must learn to remember and respect this. The art of reiki provides us with an ideal way to do this and to experience this. Once we are touched by the compassion of reiki - as I was in that hospital conference room years ago - we will never be the same again.

---

5   *Tao Te Ching*, Chapter 46, John C.H. Wu translation, Shambhala Publications.

There is an ancient teaching, "As above, so below. As below, so above." Amongst other things, this teaching reminds us of the remarkable link between the microcosm and the macrocosm. Separation and duality are truly grand illusions. And too many of us are suffering from a major case of this delusion...

On the personal, microcosmic level, the art of reiki promotes harmony and balance in many ways. Chief amongst them is by aiding in relieving stress and tension, and by doing so in helping us to avoid deeper and greater illness and imbalance. The causes of stress and tensions are not going to go away anytime soon, for any of us - the wealthiest or the most destitute of us - for we do indeed live in extremely interesting and challenging times. Preserving and promoting health and wellness for the total being is something we all are in vital need of. The compassionate art of reiki excels at making unique, cost-effective, enjoyable, and beautiful contributions towards achieving these goals. "An ounce of reiki prevention is worth many tons - and thousands of dollars - of cure." I look forward to the day when arts such as reiki are taught to children as an accepted and commonsense natural method to promote and maintain wellness and to achieve greater enjoyment from life. And check the dogma at the door if you can't see the value in this. You may be in need of some purifying and cleansing reiki for your brain, so you can think more clearly. As an American, I can actually say that this is a matter of national security for my country, given the disgrace of our so-called "health-care system," which is actually an, "if you don't have the proper social status you are out of luck and on your own" system. In other words, it is a racket, a scheme, or as my dear ole Pops would say, a "gaffe" meant to enrich a privileged few while the rest potentially rot. Well, reiki is a bit of good news -we all potentially hold the keys to better health in the palms of our own hands!

This leads us to the macrocosmic applications of this art. As the Founder knew and purposely taught and intended, the compassionate healing of reiki knows no bounds. She brings us all together through the common language of kindness, compassion, respect, and wisdom. She reminds us that at our core we are indeed all one - equal sons and daughters of the same Universal Life Force, each with our own path to follow, but doing so with the knowledge that all of our unique paths are linked, as we are all climbing the same mountain of Life. We live in a time when all of our common prosperity is linked; there is no getting around this now. Things are so intertwined, interwoven, and interdependent that even a small uprising amongst warring tribes in some distant and medieval, backwater country directly threatens the world's colossus. No longer are the weak and powerless so weak and powerless. And people everywhere are waking up to this. Of course, this alone is having a tremendous destabilizing effect in our world, as the traditional arrangements of power do not like

CHAPTER ONE: Essential Reiki Foundations

being upset or threatened. Corporate power may be superseding national and religious power at the moment - but it still does not compare to the potential of people power! This is what they are so afraid of. But it is a false fear - for have no fear, reiki is here! We love you, too.

On this world, macrocosmic level it is time for us all to grow up. We have no more time nor can we afford the petty squabbling and juvenile bickering and fighting of the past. Not with the potential that exists today for cataclysmic destruction and domination. Not with the complete wasting and reckless use of our precious and irreplaceable natural resources. And not with the violence and murder which is being inflicted upon Mother Earth. Both upon Herself, the planet, and upon all creatures trying to live in peace on this planet. Our world is dying for love, love which reiki can provide us all with.

As I say, we have no more time for any of this. If you have your head buried in the sand and think that this is alarmist talk, I would humbly encourage you to retract your melon from the hole in the ground it is planted in and open your eyes. I am no alarmist or doomsayer. I am just a humble reiki person whose eyes and heart are open, and deeply feels the screams and cries of agony of the afflicted of the world. It's to the point now that Mother Earth herself is deeply wounded and crying out for help and for love. Are we going to listen, or just sit idly and let this tragic and horrendous state of affairs continue?

When we choose to help ourselves by receiving the compassionate touch of reiki knowingly or unknowingly we are "choosing" to listen to and help the entire world. Truly, as we help ourselves to be in balance and harmony, we are contributing to the balance and harmony of the entire human race and Mother Earth, herself. Now can you begin to see what a great blessing this compassionate art is?

I hope you have enjoyed this introduction to the art of reiki and to Her basic concepts. In the rest of this book we will be going into great detail regarding the specifics of the art, with a focus on the concepts, principles, and methods which are fundamental and essential for new reiki students to learn and to know - starting with an overview of the entire art in the next chapter.

For now, let's sum up the key points of chapter one:

Summary of Chapter One

- Someone who teaches reiki is properly known as a Reiki Sensei, or a Reiki Guide, Mentor, or Teacher.
- Reiki is the compassionate touch of the love of the Universe.
- Reiki is also known as the Universal Life Force, ling ch'i, the divine light, maha para shakti, and by many other names throughout human history.
- Reiki is a perfect and pure, timeless and eternal, healing energy and force.
- Reiki is beyond all dogma and is not dependent upon any specific belief system - it is a natural, universal energy- like gravity, sunlight, radio waves, and countless other universal energies.
- Reiki simply and safely provides nourishment, support, healing, and transformation for all beings and all of creation.
- All people can benefit from reiki healing and reiki training regardless of age, social status, belief system, culture, or the like, just as all people can benefit from clean, fresh water or healthy, nourishing food.
- Usui Reiki Ryoho is the name of the system of reiki healing which was developed by the Founder, O-Sensei Mikao Usui (1865 -1926).
- O-Sensei Usui was not only the Founder of this art, he was also a Saint and an Avatar of Compassion and Healing (like a modem-day Medicine Buddha).
- The Butterfly Reiki System is a modem-day manifestation of Usui Reiki Ryoho which I have developed based upon the teaching and methods utilized by O-Sensei and his disciples.
- Nowadays there are many, many reiki styles being taught all over the world, but virtually all of them (99.99999%) are descended from O-Sensei Usui's original reiki system.
- Many of these reiki styles bear little resemblance in structure and/or intent to the great gift which O-Sensei bestowed upon the world.
- Shihan Chujiro Hayashi was a well-known and very influential disciple of O-Sensei Usui.
- He made some important and beneficial modifications to the art he learned, and taught Reverend Hawayo Takata. Shihan Hayashi was an extremely courageous and compassionate man and a great leader, in life and death.

- Rev. Takata carried on Shihan Hayashi's (and by extension, O-Sensei's) work as the first reiki teacher outside of Japan, in Hawaii; and later all over North America. Her students then brought the art to the entire world.
- Rev. Takata is thus the "mother" of virtually all reiki people in the world. She came from a very humble and challenging beginning, only to transcend it all and lead a highly successful, healthy, and happy life. She was a living reiki miracle.
- The three main aspects of Usui Reiki Ryoho are: meditation, energy healing, and spiritual healing.
- Reiki promotes regeneration, maintenance, longevity, balance and harmony, as well as tranquility – for spirit, mind, and body.
- In addition to healing, the art of reiki may be followed as a Life Path which leads to greater levels of self-realization (Samadhi/Satori/ Kensho).
- Reiki is absorbed and "digested" by the energy system in a natural process very similar to the digestion of food.
- The main actions of reiki as a healing force are: cleansing and purifying; balancing, harmonizing and vitalizing; and transforming, transcending, and empowering - for spirit, mind, and body.
- The reiki attunement is the ritual process which bestows the gift of reiki healing ability. This is the only way to "learn" reiki, and this process must be conducted by a properly trained and empowered reiki sensei/teacher.
- The gift of reiki attunement cannot be bestowed by or received from books, DVDs, websites, or from a distance - only from a live and properly trained reiki sensei in a direct line of lineage from O-Sensei Usui.
- The art of reiki is an ego-less healing art, as it is the living personification of Universal Love and Compassion.
- The "General Concepts and Principles" of the art of reiki are: Everything is Energy; All Is One, We Are One; Spirit (reiki) Commands Energy; and Thy Will Be Done, not mine (live from Higher Self).

Need I say more? I think I know the answer to that question. Keep reading to learn more about this amazing art and energy. And better yet: get thee to a good reiki sensei!

CHAPTER TWO:
The Seven Jewels of Reiki

"By being receptive, we can avail ourselves of the spiritual wealth available to us. By being open, we can receive things beyond what we ourselves might imagine."

-Deng Ming Dao

The Seven Jewels of Reiki Overview

In the previous chapter we have examined many of the general concepts and principles of both reiki, and of the compassionate art of reiki. Now we will begin to explore in more depth and specific detail just what this art is all about: what it is composed of, what you can do with it, and how one practices it.

The "Seven Jewels of Reiki" are the main core elements of the art of Usui Reiki Ryoho as it was conceived of and taught by the Founder, O-Sensei Mikao Usui, and by his immediate disciples and heirs. Nowadays, however, there are many, many reiki styles available. Thus the curriculum and specifics of these reiki styles may widely vary; as does the quality, intent, and comprehensiveness of these reiki styles. Some of these styles hew fairly closely to how O-Sensei or Shihan Hayashi or Rev. Takata taught and conceived of the art. Many do not. In fact, some are barely recognizable as being descended from the Founder's original teachings and art.

Honestly, as far as I am concerned, this is fine. The energy of reiki is extremely flexible and is above and beyond any one dogma or teaching. Thus, potential stylistic variations are theoretically unlimited. Now, this doesn't mean we should all as reiki people immediately invent and market our own reiki styles - quite the opposite, actually. All most reiki people need is to learn some good, quality, basic reiki methods and meditations and then to be disciplined about practicing and living the art every day. It's that simple.

But as I say, since human beings are diverse and human cultures and beliefs can and do vary, of course this will affect the development of reiki styles and systems. In the second volume of this series ("The Compassionate Touch of Reiki: Healing Concepts, Elements, Methods") we will explore this topic in more depth. For now it should be understood that while stylistic variations are perfectly natural and acceptable - after all, reiki is a world art now - preserving the root essence of O-Sensei's art and teachings is vital for the long-term health and proper growth of the art. For instance, if Usui Reiki Ryoho in all of its known manifestations becomes diluted and dumbed down to the point of being practiced and thought of as just another generic "energy healing" technique, just another sanitized method of "energy medicine" - then it will cease to be what it was developed as and was meant to be - which was, and is, as a path towards the development and perfection of the total being. This watering down, dumbing down, and debasement of an art can be seen in various other, older Asian arts which have been in our culture a bit longer (remember, O-Sensei passed on in 1926). Look at the state of affairs in the Chinese martial arts world, where these great ancient arts with their practical methods and illumined philosophies and teachings are thought now to be merely fancy and flashy sports, and are promoted this way. Or, as in the case of t'ai ch'i ch'uan, as something suitable only for the elderly or infirm, certainly not good or practical for the average person. Contrast this with the traditional, ancient view and understanding of these arts, which is that they are precious treasures which can preserve and enrich a person's life, and the quality of society in general, in untold ways.

So, it is very important that reiki people - and most especially reiki teachers - have a clear understanding of O-Sensei's original intent and teachings. As the art spreads and grows all over the world and begins to mature, this will help to prevent mistakes from being made and harm being done to the art. To say nothing of how this would shortchange potential reiki students. The compassionate art of reiki is still a baby on the world stage and in Her historical development as an art. Let's all do what we can to help Her grow and develop properly, so that She- and by extension, we - all may prosper. Thus, I present for you the "Seven Jewels of Reiki," the core of Usui Reiki Ryoho and of the Butterfly Reiki System.

CHAPTER TWO: The Seven Jewels of Reiki Overview

Universal Life Force (Reiki)

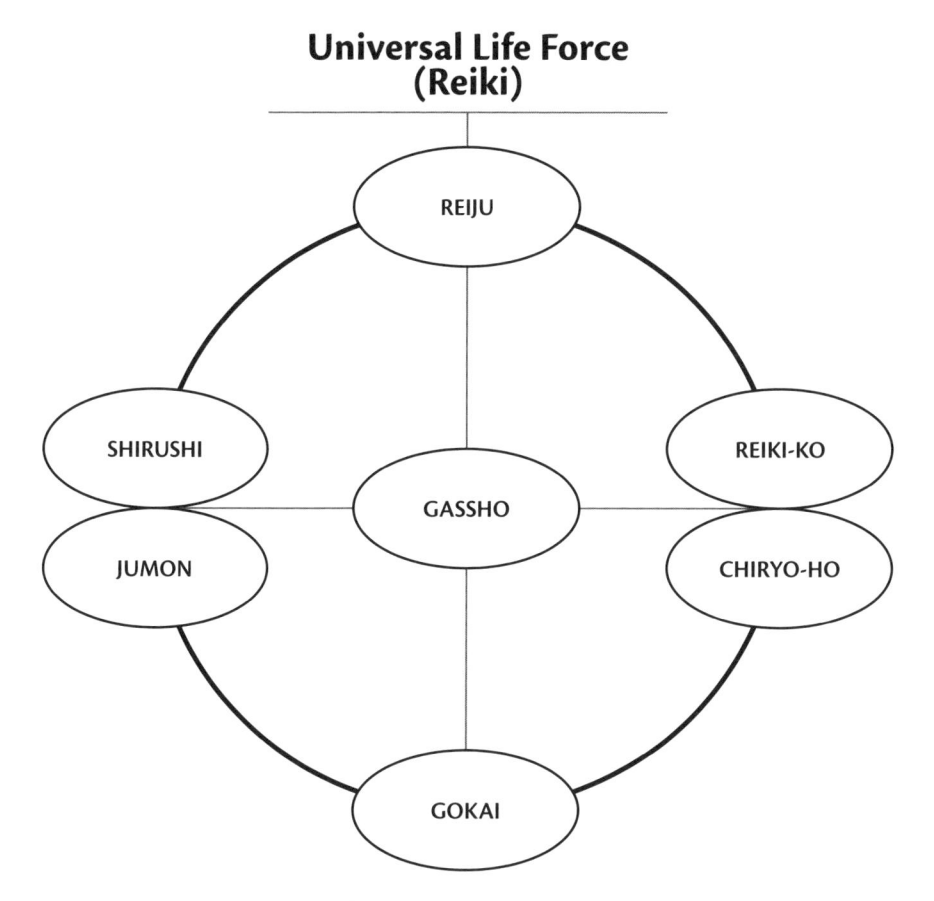

```
            REIJU
   SHIRUSHI        REIKI-KO
           GASSHO
   JUMON           CHIRYO-HO
            GOKAI
```

Diagram of the Seven Jewels of Reiki

Gassho

Gassho means to "bring the hands together," and refers to the well-known "prayer position" or as it is known in the Indian yogic arts, the "anjali mudra." Mudra refers to symbolic or ritual gestures, postures, or movements. Like when you wave your hand at someone it may mean either "hello" or "goodbye" depending on the circumstances and use of this gesture. In the context of the art of Usui Reiki Ryoho "mudra" is so important and essential it is like the Eighth Reiki Jewel, hidden in plain sight. Each of the Seven Jewels of Reiki Relies on mudra, with the cerntral reiki jewel of Gassho symbolizing mudra in general.

O-Sensei Usui, like most Asian spiritual teachers (keep in mind that Usui Reiki Ryoho is an interfaith art and not a religion), placed great importance upon the performance and understanding of this gesture. Symbolically, gassho represents reverence for and paying respect to the divinity and unity of all life and all of creation. Along with all associated qualities, such as sincerity, compassion, unity, balance, truthfulness, forgiveness, humility, and wisdom. We are meant to live life from our hearts, as a continual and never ending gesture of gassho towards ourselves and all of life and all of creation. The Sanskrit sacred word/mantra "Namaste" is a verbal/energetic expression of this gesture.

Technically, the gassho mudra helps us to unify mind and body, self and reiki. When we perform the basic heart gassho mudra we are unifying ourselves – all energies of spirit, mind, and body – with the Universal Life Force at the heart center. This, of course, is ideal as the art of reiki is an art of compassion, shared from the heart to all and with all.

The basic heart gassho mudra is made by bringing the hands gently but firmly together – palm to palm – at the heart center, in the center of the chest. The thumb and fingertips point upwards, and the joined palms touch the sternum.

There are many, many variations of this sacred gesture, some of which are quite specialized. In the Butterfly Reiki System we make use of several of these specialized gassho gestures, with the heart gassho mudra described above being the main and foundational one.

Another basic gassho mudra we make use of is made by bringing the hands to the forehead, slightly above and between the eyes. In addition to the above-described qualities associated symbolically with the heart gassho mudra, this one has the specialized meaning of a greater and higher level of acknowledgement and respect and gratitude. It is generally reserved as a way to greet and show respect to a very high Teacher, Saint, or Sage. For instance, if you were to actually be in the presence of O- Sensei Usui himself it would be appropriate to use this gesture towards him.

Technically, for reiki people, this mudra will center the self and reiki at the third eye/ajna energy zone. This energy zone is associated with intuition, knowledge, transcendence, and eternity. It is also the sign, seal, and symbol of the Butterfly Reiki System.

The other main gassho mudra gesture we make use of is to bring the "praying hands" as far directly overhead as is possible. Symbolically this is a very high way of paying respect to, acknowledging, and sharing gratitude with and towards the Universal Life Force, God, Allah, the Buddha Realm, The Great Spirit (pick your term). One might even prostrate oneself and touch the forehead to the earth after performing this gesture as a further sign of respect and gratitude.

CHAPTER TWO: The Seven Jewels of Reiki Overview

Technically and symbolically this gesture helps to bring us outside of ourselves, to shed our ego, and to be humble. In this way we invite and may be more open to receiving the blessings and gifts of the Universal Life Force.

There are also various specialized breathing and reiki energy exercises and meditations (reiki-ko) which make use of these gestures (and other gassho mudra gestures) in various ways. Additionally, these gestures may be incorporated into the process of reiki healing in various ways (see 'The Compassionate Touch of Reiki: Healing Concepts, Elements, Methods').

Thus, due to its extreme symbolic and technical importance, Gassho – as a gesture and more importantly as a Life Concept – is the central pillar and key element of the entire art of Usui Reiki Ryoho. It symbolizes, in a seed form as a gesture, the essence and intent of the entire art. Gassho, Namaste, Amen.

Reiju

"Everyone has the potential to receive the spiritual gift, uniting body and soul, a divine blessing."

-O-Sensei Usui

Reiju refers to the "spiritual gift" or "reiki blessing," which is more commonly known as the reiki attunement. As O-Sensei so eloquently describes in the quote above, all people are potentially able to receive attunement to reiki. It has nothing to do with belief, faith, or dogma, either. All aspects of the art of reiki are based upon natural laws of the Universe, it's just that science as of yet has not uncovered all of these laws. Regardless, the experience of millions of people now proves the safety and effectiveness of this art, as well as its beauty and compassion.

Again, it is the reiki attunement (reiju) which empowers one to be a reiki practitioner. In other words, quite simply, no reiki attunement = no reiki. The gift and blessing of reiki cannot be conferred upon someone by wishful thinking; nor by a vcr tape, skype, dvd, or website for that matter. Previous training in other related arts - no matter how extensive - is also no substitute for reiki attunement (this includes other energy arts, such pranic healing, ch'i gung, and the like).

And I must also reemphasize that the reiki attunement must be received from a live reiki sensei who has themselves been properly attuned to reiki and trained to do this, and is in a direct line of lineage from O-Sensei. The art of reiki is a living art, passed from individual to individual in an unbroken chain of life which began with the Founder. Now, when I say a live teacher I also mean "live and in person." The common modern phenomena known as "distant reiki attunement" is based upon a flawed understanding of the most basic mechanics and dynamics of the art, and is highly problematic. "Distant attunement" is never to be substituted for a live reiki attunement from a real, legitimate reiki sensei. "Distant attunement" may aid in transferring the intent for the potential student to receive real reiki attunement, and is also useful as a healing method similar to "distant reiki healing" - what I refer to as "Reiki Unity Healing" - but it will not result in a proper empowerment of the potential student. In other words, it is a shortcut which will not lead one to where you actually want to go. As far as reiki attunement goes, it is a dead end. And this is to say nothing of the debilitating and limiting drawbacks of not having a live teacher to instruct and guide the student in the subtleties of the art. These things require a live person! One cannot properly learn even the simplest of techniques from a website, email, phone call, dvd, or the like. Anyone who says otherwise is misinformed, ignorant, or trying to sell you what is called a "bill of goods" - something they know is worthless. Let the buyer beware.

Think of it this way: the Eternal Universal Flame via a "Universal Empowerment" and "Divine Attunement" lit O-Sensei's candle. Then he lit his students' and disciples' candles, who then lit their students' candles, and so on until the present moment and onward endlessly...

O-Sensei received this "Divine Attunement" due to his innate virtues (this includes his karma), combined with his most unusual and extreme discipline, compassion, and purity of heart and intent. Essentially he was "chosen" by the Universe/Spirit to bring this art into the world and to open the path of reiki and of reiki attunement for all people on this planet. This is why he is not only the Founder of this art, but also is rightly considered an Avatar of Healing and Compassion. By receiving and bringing this art to us O-Sensei has given us a tremendous gift, one which has led to a fundamental and positive shift and clarification of human consciousness worldwide, and will continue to do so. Thanks be to the Universe and to O-Sensei for this, as our world is in desperate need of healing and compassion. Amen.

When one receives reiki attunement three natural tendencies and abilities which we all possess become activated and vivified; and the reiki practitioner may naturally and simply and safely explore and make use of these abilities for their Highest Good and the Greater Good of all.

These three abilities and aspects of reiki attunement are:

CHAPTER TWO: The Seven Jewels of Reiki Overview

- Attunement to Self
- Attunement to Others
- Attunement to the Universe

In other words, by receiving a reiki attunement our ability to serve as a reiki channel for healing for all becomes active - for ourselves, for all beings, and for all of Creation. And it's a two-way channel - we may receive healing from any of these, or share healing with any of these. This is the meaning of "attunement."

The reiki attunement is received from the Universe (or from God or the Great Spirit, the Sach Khand or non-dual realm, the words are less important than the reality of the experience of Her) via what is known as the "sutratma" or "silver cord." This "divine electrical current" is an inner stream of divine light and energy which connects all aspects of divine light and energy to our soul, mind, personality, emotions, and energy and comes from the Highest Immortal Realm. In actuality, "we" are manifestations of this pure realm projected through the sutratma and created and living here on Earth and in this Universe and plane of existence. Thus, we are truly spiritual beings having physical experiences, not the other way around! All of the religions and spiritual and mystical teachings have their own teachings and myths and ways of presenting this truth, each in their own way. But at its core - stripped of the outer garments and dogma - they tell a similar tale.

Now, the Highest Immortal Realm is also where the reiki is coming from, to us personally through the sutratma. So via the sutratma or "silver cord" we are linked to this realm, and of course this "divine electrical current" is also a two-way street, a superhighway of divine light and love. The reiki attunement greatly opens and activates this inner connection to Source which we all have - "clearing the debris and obstructions off of the road" - so to speak. This of course may result in accelerating inner healing and evolution for all who receive a reiki attunement, no matter what stage of development they may be at. There is no one who would not benefit from or who is above reiki attunement; it's just the experience and results will differ from person to person depending on their stage of inner development and karma - what they are ready for. I know this from experiencing it myself and exploring it; and from having teachers who themselves were highly enlightened and extremely disciplined and compassionate, who received reiki attunement and benefitted from the experience and greatly appreciated it. This includes teachers of mine and students: Monks, Nuns, Priests, Saints, and Sages. They all, despite their previous attainments, greatly esteemed the reiki attunement and have the highest respect for O-Sensei. The quote from O-Sensei is thus a true fact, not merely his opinion. The words of a Sage such as O-Sensei should all be treated as pure reflections of truth, whether we understand them or not. If we are sincere, one day we will: the art reveals them to us.

Now, before we examine all of the specifics of the process of reiki attunement from a technical standpoint, I want to encourage people not to get hung up on terms and terminology. And also not to let the various outer rituals which reiki teachers utilize (which can very) confuse you. It is the end result of the reiki attunement process which matters, the rituals may vary - from very simple to complex. As they say, "the proof is in the pudding," it works, or it doesn't.

Let me use an analogy which most people will be familiar with: pizza. There are myriad ways to prepare, bake or cook, and serve pizza. The ingredients may vary widely. The cooking method, fuel, and cooking temperatures may vary. The pizza itself may come in many styles - thin crust New York style, deep dish Chicago style, Greek style, Libyan style, my Grandma from Florence's style, even California style! Red pizza, white pizza, oil pizza, even Hawaiian pineapple and spam pizza. Regardless, the end result is the same - pizza, the most perfect and delicious food on Earth. Now, we may prefer certain kinds of pizza over others, or even claim that certain kinds of pizza are not really pizza at all (have you seen people from the Big Apple and the Windy City fight over pizza?) - yet I think most of us would agree that there certainly is more than one way to prepare and enjoy pizza. I like them all - but please, no anchovies!

Regarding reiki attunement it is the same - there are many variations of the outer ritual - but the end result is the same - the student is empowered with reiki. If you are searching for the one true, original and perfect method - then good luck - as there isn't such a thing. All there is, is an attunement method which works for you and which you can utilize easily to empower your students with reiki.

I have received and experienced quite a few variations of the reiki attunement from reiki styles that are very well-known to styles that are much less known, but yet still highly esteemed. And guess what? They all work despite the differences in the outer rituals. This includes receiving reiki attunements from the Takata lineage; the Usui/Tibetan and Karuna© lineages; and from the Reiki Jinkei Do, Buddho/Enersense, and Essential reiki styles. I have also on my own, and in conjunction with friends and students, researched and practiced giving and receiving various other attunement methods, such as Hayashi and Furumoto lineage methods, "original" reiki reiju methods, and others. All of these methods work, and indeed are more alike than different. From all of this,

CHAPTER TWO: The Seven Jewels of Reiki Overview

combined with my other training and experiences, I utilize my own unique attunement method. But again, it is not so different from these others, and is just a natural reflection and outgrowth of my own unique experiences. It is not better or worse than any other method.

What receiving and researching all of these and other methods has done has given me a good picture and clear view of what reiki attunement is and is not in general. Keep in mind that reiki is a powerful and unlimited, multifaceted universal healing force. She is none other than the Universal Life Force. Therefore, due to the power and purity of the reiki energy there are potential variations in how She may be bestowed via reiki attunement rituals. And do not confuse ritual with the energy Herself.

The following are the key inner ingredients of reiki attunement:

1. The intent of the reiki energy Herself
2. The free will decision to receive reiki attunement (the student's intent)
3. The free will decision to serve as a channel or vessel for reiki attunement to happen through (the reiki sensei's intent)

These are the inner keys to receiving and bestowing the reiki attunement. Keep in mind that it is the intent of reiki to always be available to all and for all, for the Highest Good of All, as She is none other than a pure reflection and emanation of the love and compassion of the Universe (God). So when number two and three come together, number one is always there to serve, assist, and empower. It is interesting that a great and famous teacher from Palestine said much the same thing, "Anytime two gather in My name, I am there."

Again, the outer attunement rituals may and can vary. In the second volume of this series we will discuss this in more detail (The Compassionate Touch of Reiki: Concepts, Elements, Methods). For now I offer the following, which is a brief summary of some of the other important elements of reiki attunement:

1. The reiki Herself, which I mention again as without Her we have naught.
2. Asana – symbolically and technically, our use of proper posture and alignment during the attunement ritual (otherwise known as "body mechanics").
3. Bandha – "sealing" the flow of reiki within the reiki sensei in various ways, in order to direct and enhance the flow of reiki through the teacher, to enhance the attunement process; Bandha may be physical, energetic, or spiritual in nature and applications.
4. Pranayama – various breathing/energy methods which are utilized during

the attunement process in order to enhance and optimize its effectiveness.

5. Mudra – the physical gestures and movements utilized to convey the reiki and to perform the attunement ritual.

6. Shirushi and Jumon – the utilization of the reiki symbols and mantras during the attunement process.

7. Pratyahara – withdrawing, calming, and quieting the outer and inner senses; ideally one wants to operate from a place of inner stillness and one-pointedness during the reiki attunement process. Pratyahara facilitates achieving this state of mind by allowing inner and outer distractions to fall away and loosen their grip on our minds.

8. Dharana and Dhayana – concentration and meditation upon and union with the reiki Herself, and the intent of the reiki attunement process. In this way we may act as an ideal, pure vessel (as much as is possible) for the reiki to flow through in order to facilitate the reiki attunement. The sensei is the channel, vessel, and facilitator of and/or reiki attunement - not the initiator, creator, or controller of this miraculous and blessed happening. All of these steps are intended to aid the sensei in being as pure a vessel as possible - a clean channel, as it were, like a garden hose free of debris so that the water may freely flow through it. Except with reiki it is more like the sensei is the channel for the eternal and pure love, light, and power of the Universe, a beautiful melody and music of compassion, for the benefit and Highest Good of All.

9. Samadhi – blissful Unity Consciousness; this is the ideal state of consciousness for a reiki sensei to live in and operate from - the pure vantage point of the Higher Self and Soul. However, few reiki teachers truly operate from this level. This is a goal for us all to aspire to, and achieving it is dedicated to the Highest Good of All - it is not sought for selfish or egoistic reasons. And it may not be achieved if we try to do it that way, this will only lead to darkness. This is the level the most powerful and compassionate of reiki teachers (and self-realized spiritual teachers of all kinds) are operating from, and explains their great power, wisdom, and compassion. They act as pure mirrors, reflectors, and magnifiers of the Universal Life Force for all. In the specific case of this art and path - Usui Reiki Ryoho - this means primarily they serve as beacons and lighthouses of healing and compassion, radiating the light of reiki for and to all.

So this is a brief outline and description of the various elements which are involved in, and which reiki teachers make use of, in virtually all reiki attunement rituals. Please note that for a reiki sensei to properly conduct a reiki

CHAPTER TWO: The Seven Jewels of Reiki Overview

attunement ritual and attune a student to reiki, they do not need to be operating from anywhere near the highest levels which I just described. They just need to follow the steps properly and do their best. Remember: "Be Real... Be Reiki."

As to why the various reiki styles, lineages, and teachers make use of different attunement rituals and what is the significance and purpose/meaning of all of these rituals - this is a complex subject deserving of its own book to adequately do it justice. In other words, why do some attunement rituals utilize soft and natural breathing, while others may make use of a method which is like the dynamic tension breathing utilized in some martial arts? Why do some attunement rituals only utilize inner, energetic bandha - (either knowingly or unknowingly I might add, as I've noticed that most reiki teachers have almost zero understanding of the most elementary technical elements of what they are doing, beyond being able to follow the steps of the ritual properly) - while other attunement methods actually will utilize an overt physical bandha along with the energetic bandha?

Questions like this are like asking why do people wear different clothes and eat different foods all over the world. One answer is simple, because it is natural that we should do this. The other, technical answer is quite complex. So with reiki attunement rituals basically it comes down to it being natural for people to use different methods - this is why I encourage people right off here to not get hung up on little differences. It is the inner steps and keys which are important. In addition to this, there are many cultural, religious, and other similar factors which influence reiki attunement rituals. And another, often overlooked reason for differences of all kinds is that at a higher level of thinking we are all meant to learn from each other and to learn to accept and love one another despite the differences. Sort of like a life test which we all must take. So, as the French say, "Vive la difference!" And as the Vulcans from Star Trek so wisely observe and teach, "Infinite diversity in infinite combinations." Let's get over our differences, especially in as trivial a matter as reiki technique.

Again, all reiki teachers need to do is to learn an attunement method that works for them and that is effective and reliable. Keep in mind that there does not exist one "super-uber" attunement method, which is perfect for all teachers and all situations. In fact, as a counterpoint to this silliness, a truly self-realized reiki teacher may not need or make use of any outward ritual at all. All one who truly has achieved this and operates from this level needs to do is to look at a student who is ready for reiki attunement, or to touch them, or even just to think of them or dream of them. They might hand the student who is ready a glass of water and say, "drink this," and that might be the reiki attunement! And no, I am not making this up. Review the three inner keys to reiki attunement again - if one thoroughly masters everything involved with performing and utilizing these keys, and becomes a living personification of Reiki Herself, then of course such a teacher would be able to act in "mysterious ways." But, of course, teachers of this level of power and skill are almost unheard of. The rest of us - and that includes myself, and you other reiki teachers reading this - will need a good ritual to perform. But they are all fairly simple to learn, so no worries.

As for the potential student during the attunement process, their role is the passive one. They are the receiver of the gift. The main key is the intention to receive reiki attunement for one's Highest Good and for the Highest Good of All. After that, the best way to receive the attunement is to sit as if one is a child about to receive a perfect gift from the most perfect and loving Mother; completely innocently, trustingly, and lovingly.

At the least, the student just needs to try and relax during the reiki attunement. The sensei will usually assist the student in this process by utilizing some meditation or a similar method - but no drinking to relax before the attunement, please! Drunken kung fu may be a legitimate art, but "drunken reiki" is just a mess.

Now I don't present myself to you as a "Master Reiki," nor do I think of myself in this way - I haven't even mastered tying my shoelaces in the morning, so how could I honestly claim a lofty title such as this? I can't. However in my life, in addition to all of the various reiki methods I have learned and studied, I have been blessed to have learned and taught a wide variety related meditative, martial, and energetic arts. The Universe has guided me, out of her love for me, to many great teachers. I give great thanks for this. I have also been so blessed to have received darshan, satsang, shaktipat, empowerment, initiation, and teachings from a variety of self-realized spiritual teachers from a very diverse range of ancient and modem lineages and spiritual paths. All of this gives me a rather unique view of reiki, the art of reiki, and of the reiki attunement compared to the vast majority of reiki teachers and mislabeled "reiki masters" out there. You know, such as "Uncle Joe the Reiki Master" who lives down on the comer. He is a wonderful and sincere man. But after only three or four classes - he used to be a fireman, by the way, and just recently became interested in reiki to help with his stress and aches and pains, and wants to share the art with family and friends - and only a month or two of experience, "Uncle Joe the Reiki Master's" actual level of mastery is commensurate with his experience, which is almost nothing. And I say this not to disparage "Uncle Joe" or "Aunt Edna" or "my buddy John the Reiki Master" or anyone else. I say this only to point out that learning to give someone a reiki attunement does

CHAPTER TWO: The Seven Jewels of Reiki Overview

not equate to "Mastery of the Art of Reiki," even if this person has a pure heart.

This preposterous and misguided teaching and understanding of the concept of reiki mastery has led to so many problems, both with the art's public image and with the silly, egoistic squabbling amongst "Reiki Masters." Equating learning how to perform a reiki attunement with "Mastery of Reiki" is like saying that someone who knows how to put a key in a lock, open a door, walk inside a building, go up and down the stairs, and flip on and off the light switches is a "Master Architect." What would you think of someone that told you they were a "Master Architect" when actually they just knew how to get in and out of and utilize the building? They might be completely sincere and well-meaning – as are the majority of people who perform reiki attunement rituals, and I love them for this. But this would be odd, to say the least.

What I am getting at is that it is indeed true that compassion and sincerity are the keys to this art, and that includes receiving and performing a reiki attunement. But there is also no substitute for actual, real training and experience. And we all need to keep our feet on the ground in regards to these matters. I present all of this information and my experience to potential reiki students, as well as to other reiki teachers, as a gift and humbly in the spirit of being in service. This is what I am here for. Namaste.

The Seven Jewels of Reiki

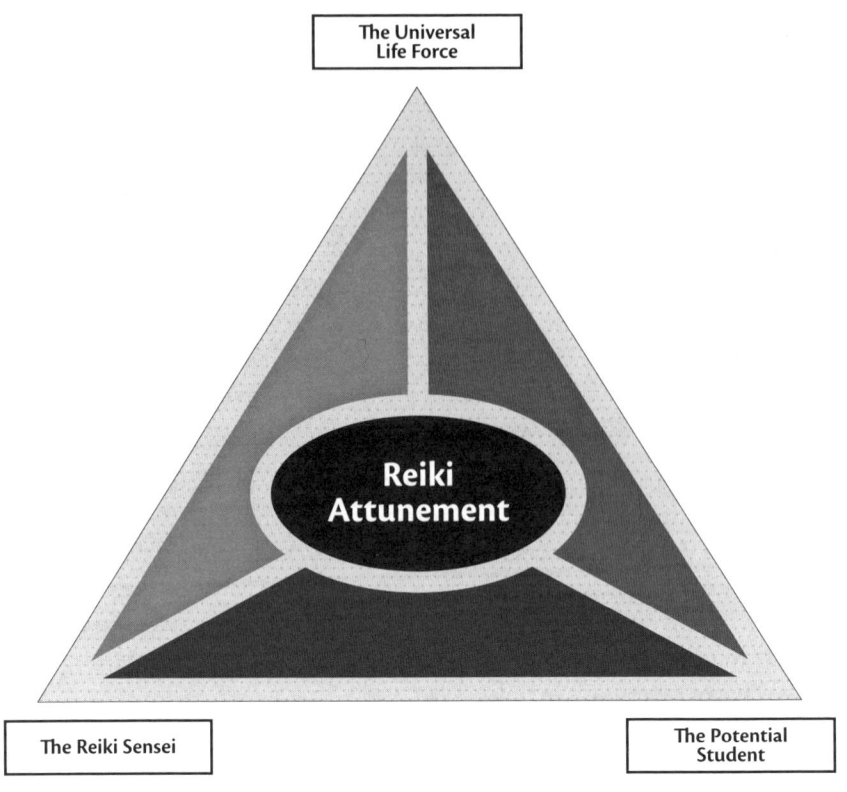

```
        The Universal
         Life Force

              △
           /  |  \
          /   |   \
         /  Reiki  \
        / Attunement\
       /_____\

The Reiki Sensei         The Potential
                            Student
```

The Inner Keys of Reiki Attunement

Gokai

"Gokai" refers to the Reiki Life Concepts, or as they are more commonly known, the Usui principles or precepts of reiki. They are like a written code or creed - a philosophy of living which O-Sensei and his disciples taught to their students in order to help them to develop themselves further as they tread the reiki path. I like to think of them as a manifestation of the gassho mudra, as they summarize the intent of the reiki path in a simple written form; as the gassho mudra does with a gesture.

We human beings tend to think too much - and to think, and think, and then to think some more. And all of this "deep thinking" doesn't always contribute to our, or anyone else's, Highest Good. Thus, with the Gokai we have something very good to contemplate and to think about - and more importantly, to live and demonstrate in our lives. This is our ultimate goal with reiki: to learn to become a living personification of the energy of reiki - Universal Love, Light,

CHAPTER TWO: The Seven Jewels of Reiki Overview

and Compassion. Thus, we must strive to "Be Real, Be Reiki."

It is very common in the Asian martial, meditative, and healing arts that the Founders and teachers of these arts share codes such as this with their students. It is far from being unique to this art. My martial arts teacher gave us several, for students and for instructors, key concepts and principles of the art. I have two from two other teachers of mine on my desk in front of me where I write, and the Gokai under a picture of O-Sensei on my wall. The codes and creeds of the various arts reflect the core essence of what the intent of the art is, and in the case of Usui Reiki Ryoho, of O-Sensei's enlightenment and understanding of the essence of how we should live as reiki people. The Founders and self-realized leaders of arts like reiki have a very clear understanding of their arts - as it may be said that indeed, they ARE their arts. Thus we should treat their words and teachings with great respect and sincerely try to always follow them, and reverently at that.

Here is a translation of the Gokai, thanks to Mr. James Deacon and his wonderful reiki resource, www.aetw.org for providing and sharing it:

"The secret method of inviting blessings, the spiritual medicine of many illnesses (Shofuku no hiho, Manbyo no rei yaku)

Just for today (Kyo dake wa):

Don't get angry (Okoru na)

Don't worry (Shin pai suna)

Be grateful (Kansha shite)

Work diligently (Gyo wo hage me)

Be kind to others (Hito ni shinsetsu ni)

Mornings and evenings sit in the gassho position and repeat these words out loud and in your heart (Asa you gassho shite kokoro ni nenji kuchi ni tonaeyo) For the improvement of mind and body (Shin shin kaizen)

Usui Spiritual Healing Method (Usui Reiki Ryoho) The founder, Mikao Usui (Chosso, Usui Mikao)"

This is a fairly literal translation of the Gokai into English. Of course, there have been many "freestyle" renderings of them as well, which still capture and convey their intent. This is a version which Rev. Takata shared with her students:

Ethical Principles of Reiki

Note that Rev. Takata was teaching reiki to North Americans in Hawaii, the mainland U.S. and Canada after WWII up to about 1980. The culture here then was quite different and "alien" compared to Japan of O-Sensei's time when and where the Gokai were born. Thus, she adjusted the translation of the concepts and principles somewhat to more properly fit the people she was working with, but preserved the original intent. All good teachers will do this, to a point.

Here is another presentation of the "Spiritual Precepts of Reiki" as presented by Rev. Takata. This is from a taped recording of a class she taught. Thanks to Ms. Earlene F. Glaeisner for sharing this, from her small but wonderful book, Reiki in Everyday Living:

Just for today, do not anger

Just for today, do not worry

We must count our blessings and honor our fathers and mothers, and our teachers and neighbors and honor our food by making no waste and show gratitude for all this also

Make your living honestly

Be kind to everything that has life

Rev. Takata's teachings are especially relevant for us, as she was the person who was chosen and trained by Shihan Hayashi – as his disciple – to bring this art to the West, and to carry on the lineage. This means so much more than merely teaching the techniques. She was chosen and trained to be an emissary, like a UN Diplomat, of the art. She had to know the art and be trained in all of its subtleties, methods, concepts, and principles. So intimately that reiki and the art of reiki was as visceral to her as her own blood and breath and heartbeat were. I find her words and teachings to literally drip with the essence of reiki, as beautiful reiki pearls and reiki jewels of light and compassion.

There is a revisionist history of the art of reiki which has been going on for some time now. In this "alternate universe" history, Rev. Takata is made out to be some sort of simpleton stooge, and the same for her teacher, Shihan Hayashi. Her teachings, such as her presentations of the Gokai, are disparaged as not "being traditional." Thus, they are thought to be tainted somehow. On the contrary, being a true innovator in an art like reiki is a hallmark of an advanced teacher. The art isn't a relic or museum trophy. It is a living art. Obviously Rev. Takata presented reiki as a life art, and more importantly, demonstrated it in her extraordinary life. Look at what she was able to accomplish despite many, so many, obstacles to her success - to her very life. To be able to overcome all of this and to transcend it as she did to become the progenitor of this art, in the lineage of the Founder and her teacher, for the entire world, is amazing! I am in awe of Rev. Takata having had many difficulties in my life, myself. But they are nothing compared to hers. She is quite an inspiration.

All of this revisionist history comes down to egoistic issues, issues related to power and control and of the deification of the self. Imagine a classical pianist and teacher who bashes the greats of his past- such as Beethoven - and those of his own time, in order to enhance his own reputation - and business. All of these modern "holier than thou" so-called "reiki traditionalists," as far as I am concerned, stink and are like a bunch of truant and disrespectful children. Some people are capable of and recognize the value of creativity and innovation. Some are not. If you are of the latter category, that is your laziness. But do not make a fool of yourself and dishonor yourself, your art, and its beautiful and loving principles or dishonor your students and your potential students; and make a mockery of the art in the general public's mind by presenting and treating this art like you are merchandizing and selling the latest microwave oven. You must be above such pettiness. "Be Real, Be Reiki."

And I realize that these are strong words. But sometimes rotten, disrespectful, and truant little children need "tough love." And by the way, none of the phonies can fool me. But no worries, we love you too. Just please, man – or woman – up! Be a real reiki person, and respect your elders, your teachers, and everyone else. Most importantly, respect yourself enough to rise above the silly pettiness of thinking you are better than other people and bashing people such as Rev. Takata and Shihan Hayashi, who are deserving of our highest respect and gratitude.

Back to the Gokai. I was taught long ago that we may learn the right way to live by observing those who live the wrong way. Not to judge them. We must love them and do what we can to help them. But we must learn from their mistakes and apply the wisdom in our own lives, just as we do by learning from our own mistakes. So, we have the beautiful concepts and teachings of the Gokai - then we have the anti-Gokai. I find it interesting that the very ones who advocate a "traditional" understanding of the Gokai as concepts to be lived in the examples of our lives - do not follow their own advice and are openly being disrespectful, very interesting. Is this what being a "reiki traditionalist" means, to be a hypocrite and to mass market your art via online "distant attunement course?" If so, I am glad that I am not a traditionalist as you are. But God Bless you, and good luck to your students.

You see some of this garbage with some of the "New Age" reiki lineages, as well; petty squabbling and egoistic posturing. If you truly are a Light Being from Atlantis - act like it!

Here is another wonderful and beautiful translation of O-Sensei's concepts and teachings from the Reiki Jin Kei Do lineage, and a very "traditional" one at that:

> Be mindful each moment of your day:
>
> To observe the arising of greed, anger and delusion, looking deeper for their true cause
>
> To appreciate the gift of life and be compassionate to all beings
>
> To find the right livelihood and be honest in your work
>
> To see within the ever changing nature of your mind and body
>
> To merge with the universal nature of the mind as reiki flows within you
>
> By following these Reiki Ideals daily, your mind and body will truly transform with the power of Reiki

And there are many others besides these, as well. Personally, I love to read and learn from all of them, as being reflections of the pure essence of reiki clarified into a linguistic verbal code, their variations are endless, like the facets of a beautiful, living reiki jewel.

These principles are so important and essential. Truly, it is our emotions which are the root cause of almost all illness. In modern medicine it is well known that stress is the cause of the vast majority of al illness and disease. This is another way of saying our emotions get us into trouble. And as we all know, "like attracts like." In other words, negative emotions such as anger and worry only serve to invite in the entire family, clan, and host of none other than our great enemy: F.E.A.R.! You know, "False Emotions Appearing Real." And as a great American President put it so eloquently: "The only thing we have to fear, is fear itself."

This is oh so true. This statement and its ramifications (along with the art of reiki) should be taught to all children as soon as they are able to begin to understand words and language; and from before then by giving all children the love they deserve and need. Love is the opposite of fear. Fear divides, love unites.

CHAPTER TWO: The Seven Jewels of Reiki Overview

Now, just as we need to love our ego and not fear him, we need to love and thank our fears. We are probably always going to have some, most of us, anyways. Regardless, we do not want them to control us. They are naught but our respected and beloved teachers, nothing more and nothing less. And fear can teach us in so many ways. For instance, we should always question individuals and organizations who are using fear to try to control and manipulate us.

You know, as in "vote for me or the world will end and Satan will take over," and similar fear-laced incentives. And in so many small ways which people utilize or fall prey to fear.

There is a place for fear in life and in teaching and learning, but only if the use of fear is dedicated to and intended for the Highest Good of All. For instance, if young Bobby keeps running into the road without paying attention to traffic, and after talking to Bobby about this – "See those cars? If they hit you, you will die. And I love you so much so I want you to be careful" – he keeps up this dangerous behavior, then it may be necessary to take further action. This is for his own good, which he is not yet capable of understanding; such as sending him to his room with no dinner, no TV, no video games, or the like. Children – and the child in all of us – need love. But sometimes some good and proper discipline is the best form of love. And I'm not talking about violence.

So as I say, we must examine fear, regardless of where it may be coming from. The fear, anger, and worry may be coming from within, or from outside ourselves. It may be completely irrational and imaginary fear, or it may fear, anger, and/or worry which has a basis in some real problem, such as chaotic and unsettled financial situations, lack of food, or worse. Regardless, we need to examine the source of the fear and its cause and do what we can to learn from, heal, and transcend it, not let it paralyze and control us. This is indeed what the compassionate art of Usui Reiki Ryoho is here for – to help us transcend our fears and realize love, life, and the opportunities we have. And I understand that unfortunately, there are many who have no opportunities in life. They are born into misery, extreme poverty, slavery, or worse. For these people we must offer ourselves and our love and service. For in this modern day and age this should not be. It does not have to be, we must agree to change this.

For those of us who, thankfully, have some opportunity in life, "Have no fear, Reiki is here!" Sorry, I couldn't resist that one. But it is the reiki version of "fear no evil." Now, entire books could be written about the Gokai, and have been. Gokai actually translates as "Five Principles." But they should be more rightly thought of as limitless Reiki Life Concepts. They are indeed simple yet profound teachings, and contain within them - in a seed form - the essence of the entire path of self-realization through the art of reiki. Such was O-Sensei's attainment that he could clarify the path down to simple and easy to understand concepts. Always sticking to them is another matter. This will take a form of practice that may be called "life's journey of discovery." Each and every one of us indeed has a unique path and journey through life. So, describing the exact way for people to learn to live the Gokai as Life Concepts, and to wisely and compassionately apply in our lives for the good of all is a challenge. We must each find our own way to do this. Regardless of how we do it, we are going to need to be mindful and vigilant for it to happen.

Another way of saying this is that we need to learn to be self-aware; in all situations and at all times. To truly live the Gokai we cannot lose our focus. Now this may sound like hard work, if you haven't learned how to properly do this, but it really isn't. It just takes some practice, some time, and soon enough you get used to it and relax into it. Then it becomes a very pleasurable activity.

So to develop awareness of self, what I recommend the most is for people to learn a very simple form of breathing meditation, such as the "Gassho Tranquility" meditation I describe later in the book or the shamatha meditations taught by various Buddhist teachers, or any similar breathing methods. There are dantien breathing methods ("chinkon") and many others. But let it be a very simple one where you learn not only to be tranquil, but to become aware of the four phases of your breath so that you can balance and heal your breathing patterns. Virtually zero untrained adults breathe properly, as small children who are healthy and animals do. The stress, pace, and misplaced focus of "modem" life literally beats the breath out of us.

The four phases of the breath are inhalation, pause, exhalation, pause. Keep in mind that "pause" is an infinitely important energetic transformational phase of the breath. It is not a mere passive void. It is the turning of Life, the eternal weaving and blending of yin and yang, or Shiva and Shakti. It is great power. For those who can achieve a certain level of self-awareness through breathe training, anyway. The breath is synonymous with life. It is so, so vital to our health, to our longevity, and to balance and harmony. When we are born, first is the breath. In life, no breath equals no life. And when we pass on, the breath of life leaves us. There is a higher, fifth phase of the breath, as well, where we learn to transcend. But start with these basics.

So, by learning to be aware of the breath through meditation, and balancing it so that it is more natural, we will derive greater health and wellness. Along with other potentials, one of which is to develop self-awareness in all situations. How, many of you may ask? Quite simply, each and every thought, each and

CHAPTER TWO: The Seven Jewels of Reiki Overview

every feeling we have, each and every action and word we utter or hear and experience – all interactions within ourselves and with the outer world and all beings – directly affects our breath. Think about it, how do you breathe when you are in love? What about when you are around someone who you very much dislike and causes you great stress, such as an abusive supervisor at work?

The truth is that everything directly affects our breath. Either subtly or in very pronounced ways – like if someone is choking you. The ancient masters knew this, as do the present day mystics and practitioners who have learned the secrets of the breath. The breath is one of the most direct links we have, and one of the most direct connecting lines we have, between the inner and outer worlds. The shamans know this, as do the true masters of t'ai chi, ch'i gung, yoga, and martial arts. It was known and taught by O-Sensei Usui as well. But many have forgotten this in the reiki world, or dropped it as it does not fit into the "fast food" model of reiki.

Developing the breath can take many years before you begin to unlock her secrets - though you will benefit right away.

So I recommend people learn some simple form of breathing meditation and practice it daily. I have practiced breathing meditation daily for over thirty years now. But I am only a beginner. I know some who have practiced for over eighty years .

The next step is to pay attention to your breath in your life. How do you breathe when you wake up? What about before bed? At work? On the drive home from work? What about with your friends? And how does that compare to how you breathe when you are with your children? Or at the movies? Around people you love? Around those who cause you obvious stress or whom you may dislike?

So, we begin to learn to be aware of how we breathe in all situations. Then we can learn to balance and improve our breath in all of these situations. We never want to have irregular, constricted, held, short, or stunted breathing. It is not healthy and will cause numerous illnesses and shorten our lives. Breathing must be natural.

In the case of living the Gokai, this has direct applications. If I am in a situation that is stressful to me, I can pay attention to it and correct my breathing. It is very hard to be angry or worried if one is breathing deeply, fully, and rhythmically. At the least doing so will take the "edge" off of these unhelpful feelings. At the same time, we can apply some compassionate thinking to the situation. If someone is being, for no reason, rude and aggressive with you (but not violent), breathe deeply and remember that we all make mistakes and we all have bad days.

There are too many ways to apply this in life for me to illustrate here. We can address specific situations as they arise. Additionally, I recommend taking a "Higher View" in general, to live from Higher Self. One way to do this, but it must be done sincerely and with no ego or vanity involved, is to view people (and ourselves) as innocent little children. Innocent children may make many mistakes and do silly or cruel things, out of ignorance. As an adult I cannot punish an innocent young child (such as a three or four year old) too harshly nor should I judge them harshly. They are too young for this, they do not know any better. And judgment and anger will not help in the end anyway. So I view all as little children, and try to be helpful and understanding and compassionate; as an adult guiding and teaching children should. If "punishment" is needed, then it is never to be done out of anger or violence or frustration. The "punishment" is only meant to educate, or to keep people from hurting each other or themselves. This may be in the form of a self-realized employer who treats her employees respectfully and values them and has compassion for them. But also holds them to their responsibilities. Or this may be applied by each and every one of us in numerous ways. But it takes a very well-balanced and mature and ego-less person to live from this state of consciousness. Thus, the first method - deal with situations as they come and mollify them compassionately by adjusting the breathing and doing what needs to be done to gracefully deal with the situation - is a good first step, which can lead to living from Higher Self all the time.

Another strategy of living the Gokai is to apply the teaching of karma. Quite simply, if you are open to the concept of karma - or as it says in the Christian Bible, "As ye sow, so shall ye reap" - and to the possibility of reincarnation (which is merely an extension of the concept of karma) then this approach may work. And that is to understand that since time is eternal and that reality has no boundaries - there are an untold numbers of Universes, dimensions and sentient beings - each and every one of us has been at one time the mother, brother, sister, father, and child of everyone else. We all have been each other's murderers, torturers, co-workers, strangers, as well - we have all been in every kind of relationship that is possible with everyone we meet and deal with in life. Given this truth - which cannot be denied if we are open to karma and reincarnation - we should develop the view and understanding that all people and all beings are our loving Mother. And we should love them as such. So, even when Mom does something we may not like, she is still Mom and we still love her, right? Even if Mom committed crimes that sent her to jail, she would still be our mother, the one who gave us life. Even an abusive mother

CHAPTER TWO: The Seven Jewels of Reiki Overview

must be forgiven, as it is possible to do so, and loved for having given us the precious gift and opportunity of human life.

So, these are some ideas on how to develop one self and some related strategies for how to live the Gokai as Life Concepts each and every day of our lives. I cannot overemphasize how important having an experienced teacher is, one who has been through and mastered the concepts, methods, and applications that we are trying to learn. Having such a teacher is a priceless opportunity, one worth climbing mountains and crossing deserts and oceans for. Seek well young grasshopper.

Please note: the methods I am describing are not meant to be substitutes to or for medical or psychological evaluation or treatment. They are what they are, and may be practiced by all, in conjunction with whatever other therapies that may or may not be needed.

There is much more I could say relating to Gokai and living the Concepts of the Gokai. But for now, let me simply say: living in the present moment - the eternal here and now - and not being controlled by our past or fearful of our future, whilst we bow in reverence to and with gratitude and love for all; as we release, learn from and transcend our angers, worries, and fears - is truly the way we are meant to live and to walk and share the path of reiki with others. Namaste and great thanks to O-Sensei for sharing this blessed teaching with us.

"Reiki is Wisdom and Truth."

-Rev. Hawayo Takata

Reiki-ko

Reiki-ko is the art of reiki energy work, or reiki ch'i gung (qigong). Of the seven core elements of the art of Usui Reiki Ryoho, this is the one that has most often been left out, forgotten or glossed over, nowadays. A large percentage of reiki people have never even heard of reiki-ko, or reiki meditation and reiki energy work. The main reason for this is that reiki-ko is resistant to a "fast food" approach to learning and teaching reiki. Like all meditative or yogic methods, reiki-ko must be practiced regularly and for years to achieve even a basic level of skill and understanding, though of course the reiki student begins to benefit from such practice right off.

This is the same for all arts, crafts, and disciplines, as well; music, singing, sports, basket weaving, what have you. They must be learned from someone with a demonstrated level of skill, and then practiced by the student to achieve anything or to get anywhere with them. There are very few inborn, natural geniuses amongst us who are able to teach and guide themselves right from the beginning. Even Michael Jordan was cut from his high school basketball team! He needed to learn to focus his mind and intent and take practice seriously. This, combined with his natural, inborn gifts, led him to become one of the greatest basketball players ever to live, and an international icon of success. And yes, the second year he tried out for his high school team he did make the cut! I could give you many more examples like this of people with great inborn skills and talents that still needed to practice and persevere to achieve success. And it is the same in all fields. In fact, this is perhaps the most overlooked key to true mastery and success - it takes discipline. The day after Larry Bird won his first NBA title he showed up unannounced at 6:00 a.m. at a teammate's house so that they could go for a long run and begin training for the next season! Now that's discipline.

I was at a martial arts seminar a few years ago with a well-known leading Filipino martial arts master in my country here, himself a student and disciple of a legendary and pioneering Filipino Grandmaster. Another more inexperienced student asked this teacher what his teacher did to become so wildly skillful at his art. He thought there must be some "secret technique" and wanted to know it. But the teacher, who is very honest and pragmatic, gave him the straight truth. He told this young student that if you saw the real masters practice, you would be greatly disappointed. It ain't like in the movies, you know, like Buckaroo Banzai. All the masters do is practice day after day and year after year, so that they may thoroughly embody the basics of their art and then transcend them so they can be applied in all situations. That's it. Just practice hard every day and be creative with it. Indeed this is the real meaning of "kung-fu" - a high skill which has been developed through time and much effort. There is no other way. I give great thanks that I was taught this "secret" by my teacher from moment one upon meeting him.

Well, of course O-Sensei Usui knew this and taught this as well. Originally reiki was taught in a dojo type of setting - in a school where students practiced under the direct supervision of highly skilled, trained, and experienced teachers. And of course reiki-ko was something that they practiced regularly, in every session and at home. Keep in mind that while reiki attunement does indeed impart the great gift of reiki and reiki healing ability to all - it only confers the potential to have skill within the various reiki sub-arts, such as reiki-ko and reiki chiryo-ho (the actual reiki healing methods.) For us to truly develop any skills or achievements with these we must practice and practice well. Remember: practice makes perfect. And discipline leads to freedom. This

CHAPTER TWO: The Seven Jewels of Reiki Overview

is a truth we must all confront at some point on the reiki path.

As I have already mentioned, before I came to reiki I had been learning, practicing, and teaching daily a wide variety of from the meditative, martial, and healing disciplines, and with a spiritual perspective under the guidance of some extraordinary teachers. My second reiki teacher was a highly gifted and real clairvoyant, as she demonstrated for all to see many times. In my second reiki class with her, her husband was in attendance and was my practice partner. He happened to have a mild knee injury at the time. Well, I had also been reading about and studying "color healing" a bit back then. So I decided to try and combine the color healing with the reiki, and accessed and visualized a beautiful, vibrant and warm, emerald green healing energy to give the reiki some "color." I wanted to experiment with how this would affect the applications of reiki healing.

Well, from across the room my teacher noticed what I was doing and commented, "I think that green energy you are giving him is helping his knee, keep it up!" I was flabbergasted that she knew this. There is no fooling or playing games with this woman - as she can clearly "see" people's thoughts and feelings, as well.

Now, I mention this because this same talented and powerful reiki teacher told me, in my first class with her, that because of my previous years of experience and discipline with various other energetic arts (ch'i gung, t' ai chi, meditation, kung-fu, yoga) that I was already internally cleansed to the point that even as a brand new reiki student the reiki was already flowing through me more easily and more strongly than in most reiki teachers with years of experience. This was something that she could actually see, it was not a guess. To me it was just natural back then, but now I understand the implications of what she told me very well. This lady was also the first to help me understand what my "mission" on Earth in this life was, and helped me in so many ways. I can't thank her enough and love her greatly, she is like my reiki Mommy. Interestingly enough, it is actually Mother's Day here as I sit and write this.

Now, I mention these things not to toot my own horn but as a vivid and personal example of the great importance and value of practicing reiki-ko. Even one or two simple methods practiced regularly can transform someone's reiki practice and inner health and balance, taking them to an entirely different and higher level. Think of it this way, if one wants a healthy and strong body then one must exercise regularly. Well, if you want a healthy and strong and balanced inner flow of energy and reiki, then you must practice reiki-ko. This is why it can be called "reiki exercise."

And these two are linked and support each other, our inner and outer levels of health and balance. We should not ignore either or favor one over the other.

Essentially, reiki-ko consists of a variety of specialized forms of reiki meditation, reiki breathing exercises, and reiki energy exercises. And there can be quite a bit of diversity here. The main reasons for practicing reiki-ko are as follows:

- greater ability to focus and unify mind, body, and reiki
- practice aids in achieving even deeper levels of inner peace and tranquility
- practice will aid in purifying, cleansing, and strengthening the reiki student's entire energy system

These foundational benefits of Reiki-ko practice may lead to the following benefits:

- enhanced personal health, vitality, and longevity
- balance and harmony of all aspects of being - spirit, mind, and body
- greater spiritual clarity and tranquility

All of this may lead to:

- being cleaner and clearer channels for reiki healing energy
- increasing and expanding our reiki skills and abilities

Which may lead to:

- greater ability to heal ourselves, achieve happiness, and to share the gift of reiki with others
- thus, Reiki-ko practice is a compassionate, win-win blessing!

So, as you can see, reik-ko practice is a very important and unique element within the proper practice of the compassionate art of Usui Reiki Ryoho. And the same goes for the proper and well-rounded development of the reiki student. And that means all of us reiki people, by the way. We must all always be students, or else we are nothing.

Now, basically, reiki-ko is just a more subtle and ingenious method of applied reiki healing, a potentially and virtually unlimited one. In other words, it is reiki healing, like putting your reiki hands on yourself or someone else is reiki healing. It's just another, more subtle way of doing it. Some of the reiki-ko exercises will be practiced from a seated position, some from a standing position, and some may be practiced lying down (front, side, or on the back.) Some are still in nature – no body movements, while others involve body movements of various kinds.

Now, as we have discussed and reiki people know, it is the reiki attunement which bestows the gift of reiki and reiki healing ability. Reiki-ko is one of the traditional reiki sub-arts which was taught by O-Sensei and his disciples. Arts which are similar to reiki-ko include: shinki-ko, ch'i gung and nei gung, pranayama, kundalini, and kriya yoga, and Min Zin - amongst others.

When a skilled, knowledgeable, experienced, and intuitive teacher of any of these arts combines them with reiki attunement and reiki energy, it is possible to develop and create unique Reiki-ko methods. After all, we are the vessel for the reiki energy. The expression of reiki energy via reik-ko methods is thus virtually unlimited. Within the Butterfly Reiki System, in addition to the traditional reiki-ko methods of Usui Reiki Ryoho (which I have updated a bit), I have also developed and adapted for the practice of reiki various relevant and essential reiki-ko methods from my own unique experiences with related arts. This development has been taken under the guidance of some quite remarkable teachers, as well, with their input and advice. These are people who have the highest quality world-level training and experience and have been at it much longer than I have been alive. Nothing related to the Butterfly Reiki System is something which has been developed in some haphazard, careless, or disjointed fashion. It all has connections and comes from real time-honored and tested and proven traditions - some quite ancient - and I have been developing this system myself since 1997. Later in the book the foundational B.R.S. reiki-ko methods will be listed and examined.

Again, one doesn't necessarily need to learn a huge list of these methods. Even one or two good methods practiced regularly will yield results. I have developed a very comprehensive and well-rounded reiki system, but don't let it intimidate you. People will practice what they need to benefit, and we are all different. "In the flowering beauty of springtime, some of the branches will grow long, and some short." This is only natural.

Also, ideally one should learn reiki-ko from someone with at least three years of daily personal experience practicing whatever they are teaching you; and someone who has learned from someone else in this way (not from a book, dvd, skype, or website). This is so that sidetracks, pitfalls, and mistakes do no happen. Even the simplest reiki meditation and reiki-ko methods should be learned this way. Missing the mark by even a small amount can lead one miles away. Reiki-ko practiced well is a great blessing. Practiced improperly it can be deleterious to health and quite damaging, even to the point of death. Imagine the damage which could be done if someone improperly learned a breathing method, and then practiced it with great zeal. This could actually cause harm. So learn from someone who is experienced and grounded. And enjoy, when you practice Reiki-ko you are giving yourself and the world a great gift. Congratulations! For more on reiki-ko and qigong in general see both the second volume on reiki in this series, The Compassionate Touch of Reiki: Healing Concepts, Elements, Methods; and my book The Shaolin Butterfly Style: Art of Transformation.

> "The reward in a thing well done lies in having done *it*."
>
> -Ralph Waldo Emerson

Jumon and Shirushi

> "And God said, 'Let there be Light,' and there was Light."
>
> **-Genesis**

Before we discuss the next two reiki jewels individually, I would like to address them together with some general commentary. And since in the art of reiki the jumon (or "reiki mantras") and the shirushi (the reiki "symbols") are generally utilized simultaneously this is only appropriate. They go together like peas and carrots – or as in spiritual light and sound do, as the quote above suggests.

First some definitions:

Mantra- (Sanskrit: Mantra, literally "instrument of thought" for man, to think) – A sacred text or passage, especially from one of the Vedas used as a prayer or incantation. Also a holy name for inward meditation.[6]

> "Mantra is a Sanskrit word with many shades of meaning: 'tool of the mind,' 'divine speech,' and 'language of the human spiritual physiology' are just a few of these."
>
> - Namadeva Thomas Ashley-Farrand

Jumon - spell; charm; incantation; magic word[7]

---

6   The Oxford English Dictionary, 2nd Ed.
7   Jeffrey's Japanese English Dictionary

CHAPTER TWO: The Seven Jewels of Reiki Overview

Kotodama - literally "word spirit/soul"; English translations: "soul of language"; "spirit of languages"; "power of languages"; "power word"; "magic word"; "sacred sound"

Symbol - a written character or mark used to represent something; a letter, figure, or sign conventionally standing for some object, process, etc.[8]

Yantra - (Sanskrit: Yantra, literally "a device or mechanism for holding or fastening") - a geometrical diagram used as an aid to meditation in tantric worship; any object used similarly[9]

-Note: "Tantric worship" does not necessarily only mean "tantric sex," as there are many tantric paths, arts, and methods besides the tantric sexual arts. Indeed, the art of reiki may be viewed and practiced as a tantric art. Don't forget that "sex sells" - even in the spiritual world! There are many charlatans out there leading "tantric sex workshops," which are really none other than "spiritual sex toys," batteries included. Let the buyer beware, as some of these are quite harmless diversions, but some may be dangerous. It isn't meant to be a game or an exotic form of hedonism, but actually a path to enlightenment.

Shirushi- sign; symbol; indication[10]

Alright, now let's examine just what we are talking about here. Unfortunately, these two elements within the art of Usui Reiki Ryoho, jumon and shirushi, seem to have been misunderstood by a great many reiki teachers and reiki people out there. Let's try to shed some light on this subject:

Since ancient times within the vast panoply of meditative, healing, and spiritual arts and disciplines the use of mantras and symbols for all manner of purposes has become a quite intricate and well-developed art and science. In fact, one could devote one's whole life to this study and still fall far short of learning all that there is to learn. They are exceedingly deep and comprehensive arts and disciplines.

Additionally, this art and science has permeated all aspects of society - witness the omnipresent "golden arches" symbol and the mantra "you deserve a break today!" The Nike swoosh-Just do it! And the (formerly) almighty $ - the buck stops here! From religions and governments, to business, marketing, and advertising, to politics and sports, virtually no area of life is untouched by this ancient, universal discipline. Who can forget Adolph Hitler's perverted

---

8 The Oxford English Dictionary, 2nd Ed.
9 The Oxford English Dictionary, 2nd Ed.
10 Random House Japanese-English, English-Japanese Dictionary

and evil use of the swastika - the symbol of spiritual victory - for his sick and twisted dystopian vision of the Third Reich? Or, in a more positive example, the use of the song "We are the World" as a symbol and mantra for so many noble causes? And it's true, by the way - it's up to me and you to make a better day! Ahh, I love that song...

O-Sensei Usui, the Founder, was an extremely gifted, disciplined, and experienced individual - both in life and in the various meditative, martial, and healing arts of his culture - and of many cultures. Therefore, it is quite natural and makes perfect sense that he incorporated the use of jumon and shirushi into his art. Given that Usui Reiki Ryoho is meant to be easily learned and practiced by all people - rather than say, only by Brahmin Priests, Buddhist Scholars, or Vedic Pandits - the use of symbols and mantras in this art is relatively simple. This is also due to O-Sensei's brilliance that he was able to develop a simple system which is still comprehensive, effective, and without limitation. Take a look at some of the traditional and mind bogglingly complex Hindu or Tibetan rituals and systems which use mantra and symbols and you will see what I mean. Some of them may take weeks, months, years, or even lifetimes, to complete.

In fact, it is generally accepted that O-Sensei taught only four symbols and their accompanying mantras. These traditional Usui reiki mantras and symbols are quite diverse and are applicable to virtually unlimited situations and applications. They aid in the creative and flexible use of this art, and help to lead the reiki student into the deepest, highest, and most subtle and esoteric aspects of the art and Her applications. Thus, they are true "reiki power tools." As such they are empowered aspects of the Universal Life Force which utilize the vibratory/sound and light principles of the Universal Life Force in order to aid in concretizing, or bringing to life, all potential applications of the art of reiki. Thus, we are co-creators with the Universal Life Force, and the jumon and shirushi are two of the main paints and paintbrushes we utilize to create our beautiful reiki art with. And as always, following the way of the art, which is that all is dedicated to the Highest Good, Thy Will be Done, not mine.

Of course, as reiki has spread like a fire of love and light all over the globe now, O-Sensei's original art and teachings have undergone evolution, transformations, and alterations. This is only natural and it is not to be feared. Everything changes, everything is undergoing constant transformations - and the art of reiki is a living art, it is not a relic to be placed on a pedestal in a museum for us to marvel over. You know, as in, "Wow! That's some nice reiki over there hanging up on the wall."

CHAPTER TWO: The Seven Jewels of Reiki Overview

"But what do you do with it?"

"Ah - I forgot, but it sure is cool, isn't it?"

So, and I say this understanding that those with more rigid ways of thinking are not going to agree, but as far as I am concerned tradition for tradition's sake alone - with no understanding of what the purpose of tradition is - leads to ossification. A reiki person told me once that you had to wear purple when you practice reiki. I responded that actually I don't, but if you have to, then go ahead. Another one told me you could only stand on the left side of someone when you give them reiki - same response, you may need to, but I don't! Now, this goes for what I call the "Pure Reiki Elite" camp as well. In fact, I just received an email from a seemingly well-meaning reiki teacher who wants to enlist my help in trying to "educate" the reiki community and promote his view and version of the art as being the "One True Way" that everyone should view and teach and practice the art. Talk about hypocritical, he criticizes all these other groups for not following the "original teachings" which he claims to have - but the thing is, O-Sensei himself taught different people in different ways according to their ability to understand and apply his teachings. This is what all the great teachers do. So what is the original teaching? People are confusing the outer garments for the essence. We live in a fast-food world, which has so thoroughly colored our thinking that it is to the point that people don't even realize it now. So, we have people come to the "reiki drive through window" and order some "reiki" and the person/teacher (or website) answers, "would you like Traditional, Takata, Hayashi, New Age, Tibetan, or today's special, Hot Sake Reiki?" And then they sell the customer their chosen brand of reiki. And these different reiki "fast food purveyors" then fight each other over who has the better product, like fast-food restaurants do - including lawsuits and ridiculous and dishonorable behavior.

So, and this is my belief, I understand that the rigid thinking or the reiki salesman are not going to agree (as they don't want thinking and understanding, they want you to buy their reiki product or join their cult) - as long as the root essence, the root principles, the root energy, and the root methods are preserved as they were transmitted by the Founder, then the evolution and transformation of the art is quite natural and acceptable. Even desirable, as it keeps it fresh and alive - in my humble opinion, anyway. And by the way, I am on a quest for the "magic super pizza," the original pizza - and when I find it I expect you all to buy it and eat it and to acknowledge its greatness - just kidding. The seven jewels of reiki are these root teachings, principles, methods, and energy. It's just that their manifestations as reiki styles is flexible, not rigid. Do not confuse the menu for the food, or the reiki style for the essence of reiki!

Now, as far as jumon and shirushi goes, this means that there are many more reiki symbols and mantras in use today by reiki people than there were in O-Sensei's day. This is just natural. But of course, more isn't always better. In general I believe we should choose quality over quantity every time with reiki. There actually is no need for more reiki symbols and mantras beyond what O-Sensei shared with us, as they are each distinct and omni-applicable. Simplicity is very close to Nature and to perfection. Keeping this in mind then, understand that it is also possible for one who has truly ascended to a very high level in this art (or someone extremely gifted and sensitive) to virtually dispense with symbols and mantras altogether. After all, they are only tools - respected and wondrous tools - but only tools. They are not the Universal Life Force. There are many tools which we may utilize to receive and transmit the Universal Life Force with. Mantras and symbols just happen to be very natural to us human beings due to our own innate virtues and makeup - they are natural extensions of body, speech, and mind.

Think of the great chefs and cooks of the world whom you may know or have seen. Do they need or are they stuck with only one recipe or one menu? No, not at all. They have thoroughly mastered their craft to the point that they have transcended the recipes. They may still consult recipe books and learn more as no one has all the answers - but essentially they have become the creators of recipes, no longer bound to strictly following the recipe on the box of macaroni and cheese. As Emeril would say, bam! Now let the music play...

Now, as "reiki chefs and reiki cooks" unless and until we become great at reiki and master it, like Emeril LaGasse has cooking, we should just stick with the use of the reiki mantras and symbols as well as the other elements of the art as we have learned them. Making stuff up is not actually helpful, it may be fun, but...

We may think of the energy and art of reiki as a great, limitless, cosmic circle. Within this great circle lie all the aspects of being, life, and of creation. This includes healing and all related to healing and transformation. The reiki mantras and symbols which O-Sensei gave us are a way for us to begin to learn to access and work with the various facets of healing contained within this great cosmic reiki circle. Beyond the simple hand positions, that is; which are by themselves quite effective and need no reiki mantras or symbols. Remember - the reiki mantras and symbols are not the energy, they are merely what I call "reiki power tools." Do not confuse the clothes for the person, or the technique for the reiki.

So, as they are merely tools - they are not the way, they are not the path, and they are not the Universal Life Force Herself- it is possible for so-called "non-traditional" (non-Usui) reiki symbols and mantras to exist, and to be safe and effective, at that. The Universal Life Force as well as mantras and symbols all existed long before O-Sensei Usui, after all.

For those who fear that this will lead to "non-reiki" forms of reiki or that this somehow negatively impinges on what anyone else is doing with reiki - you know like, "look at her! She's wearing bright fancy clothes, she is going to ruin it for us purists in our black and white uniforms!" - I would encourage you to open your minds and to employ your principles - "Have no fear - Reiki is here." Calm down, everything is going to be alright, listen to some Bob Marley, mon. Chill! Reiki as in the Universal Life Force existed before the human race did and will long after we are gone. This is the bottom-line truth. Also, different methods for accessing and utilizing the reiki existed before O-Sensei, during his time, and do today and will tomorrow.

This includes the use of different (non-basic Usui) mantras and symbols. The difference - and the great beauty, strength, and blessing - with O-Sensei's art is that now WE ALL may easily receive the blessing of reiki and of reiki healing ability, via the simple yet profound baptism of reiki attunement. It is no longer only reserved for the elite: the super-talented, the ultra-disciplined, those born into the proper caste, or the Saints and Sages amongst us, only.

O-Sensei was given a gift which he then gave to the entire world - a simple but safe, practical, and beautiful method which all may benefit from. Amen and hallelujah for that!

So, just as new reiki and reiki chiryo-ho methods can be developed, it is possible for non-Usui reiki mantras and symbols to be utilized and developed. Such as the ancient and revered Om/Aum, which many reiki people make use of.

Utilized within the context of Usui Reiki Ryoho - given they are true, authentic Universal reiki mantras/symbols as Om obviously is - they will only access and make use of the pure Universal Life Force. If we are conditioned to only seeing red roses, upon viewing a yellow rose for the first time we may be a bit perplexed, even startled. But upon inspection we will be exhilarated by our discovery. The potential beauty and diversity of reiki is like this. Many reiki flowers exist in nature, waiting to be discovered.

Now, here comes the grounding caution: The use of mantra and symbol within the art should not be taken lightly, or in a "willy-nilly" fashion. It isn't a game, like finger painting with reiki or something like this. Without the proper expert training and many years of experience both with reiki and in the mantric/symbolic sciences it is best for people just to utilize the mantras and symbols which O-Sensei gave us. If you can barely stand and walk you should not attempt to fly a spaceship, as the results may be disastrous for all involved. Leave flying the spaceship to the true cosmonauts and Captain Kirk!

Unless we have achieved this high level of skill, and a comparable level of consciousness - one comparable to O-Sensei himself - then we shouldn't "monkey around" with the art. And we must be honest with ourselves. The voice of the ego can be very seductive and tricky - but it may be a voice which is quite delusional and far from the truth. Extremists and "purists" of all stripes do many crazy things and many times wrongly thinking it is justifiable, as if God wants us to kill in his name! Do not be a reiki extremist or reiki egoist, be honest with yourself and others, be humble, "Be Real, Be Reiki." I sure haven't come anywhere close to O-Sensei's level. I know that. This isn't a criticism; I love myself all the same. It is what it is.

The only caveats I would add here is that it is possible (though rare) to learn from teachers who are both extremely advanced with meditative healing arts which make use of mantras and symbols, and are also extremely advanced with the art of reiki. These people are rare, but they do exist. To my great, good fortune I happened to meet one of these teachers, and he loves to teach and share, with great enthusiasm. I have also worked with daily and studied mantra/symbols and their uses for over thirty years now. So, the Butterfly Reiki System does indeed contain within it some "non-traditional" reiki mantras and symbols, some of which are unique to B.R.S. But the Usui mantras/symbols are at the heart of the system. The others are only reserved for those who practice well and are ready to learn more. I am not interested in creating a separate "menu" to be sold through the "reiki drive-thru." I teach one art, it just happens to be exceedingly comprehensive and deep (as far as reiki styles go, anyway). I am like the reiki/internal arts/martial arts equivalent of Scotty from the old, classic Star Trek TV show.

Remember him? Even when he was given time off, or "shore leave," he would rather spend his spare time reading and studying (and enjoying) engineering manuals. Sad to say, but I am the reiki version of this guy. Man, I need a vacation! And I am just joking. I am blessed that what I love is also what I do. What could be better?

The other caveat is that there have been reiki teachers and students - highly sincere and pure-hearted ones - who have in various states of meditation/higher consciousness been visited by spiritual beings or the Universal Life Force herself, and been given reiki mantras and symbols for them to utilize and share with others. The mantras/symbols (if they are true ones) are actual manifestations of the Universal Life Force, so this is entirely possible and does happen.

But don't forget that, unfortunately, there are also less sincere and pure-hearted reiki people out there who just make stuff up for various reasons - such as for making lots of money, and/or glorification of their bloated and deluded egos. So, even in the spiritual/healing arts world, we must not forget that these things happen, "let the buyer beware." The parting words of a very high spiritual teacher from South Africa still ring in my ears from the last time I saw her, "be vigilant!" Vigilance and wariness are different than fear, as long as we don't tinge them with fear. They are natural facets of being awake.

In my next book 'The Compassionate Touch of Reiki: Healing Concepts, Elements, Methods" we will explore the jumon and shirushi and their basic uses in great detail and depth. This includes their exact nature as classes of mantras/symbols - what makes them tick, why they work - which I haven't seen (only partially) anywhere else.

For now let's focus our attention on jumon and shirushi individually a bit more, but in a general sense.

Jumon

The Japanese word "jumon" refers to the "names" of the reiki symbols, as many reiki people know them. They are a tool which uses sound vibration in order to access and utilize the Universal Life Force known as reiki, and generally in tandem with their accompanying symbol (the "shirushi"). How this is done technically we will explore in my book "The Compassionate Touch of Reiki: Healing Concepts, Elements, Methods.

In Japan one of the ancient sciences which utilizes sacred sound is called kotodama. Various religions, spiritual paths, and teachers each have their own systems of kotodama, such as: Shinto, Omoto-kyo (Onisaburo DeGuchi), O-Sensei Morihei Ueshiba (a disciple of DeGuchi who created his own system), and reportedly O-Sensei Usui himself. Nowadays some reiki teachers even use the term kotodama for the names of the Usui reiki symbols, though in my humble opinion this is incorrect and misleading. Japanese kotodama systems are more like the seed sound mantras of Indian systems. They make use of simple but powerful seed mantras - such as o, su, ah - in order to achieve various results or states of consciousness. But the "names of the reiki symbols" are not seed sounds, they are a bit more complex in character and energy, though on the very simple side compared to the "freight train" mantric formulas, as Namadeva Thomas Ashley-Farrand calls long, complex mantric formulae. In fact, the ancient Sanskrit/Vedic scriptures in their entirety are rightly considered to be hugely complex mantric formulations. So the Usui mantras are simple, but they are not single-seed kotodama. My understanding is kotodama technically may have up to three syllables and are very simple but pure and powerful - like oh, ah, ooh - but still the Usui mantras are a bit more developed than kotodama (two are and two are not). So, the terms jumon or mantra are a bit more accurate for the Usui "names of the symbols" as many reiki people know them.

Now, if an actual, verifiable, authentic and complete kotodama system from O-Sensei Usui is brought forth and someone with sufficient training and skill were to share this with us, then that would be excellent and most interesting. But I haven't seen or heard of this yet. All there is at this point is bits and pieces of "reiki kotodama" out there, presumably derived from the writing and teachings of O-Sensei Ueshiba - not from the Founder of our art, O-Sensei Usui.

For instance, the kotodama for the Usui reiki symbol known as C.K.R is said to be: o u eh ee. I find this interesting and have experimented with positive results with these Usui kotodama, and am eager to learn more. But for now, until an actual authentic and coherent system is presented - not just bits and pieces culled from who knows where - I stick with the jumon and shirushi as I have learned them. After all, they have worked for millions of people all over the world since O-Sensei shared them with us. There is no need to rush to reinvent the wheel, when the wheel isn't broken.

Kotodama as a system, though seemingly simpler, is actually more difficult for the average person with little or no meditative background to make use of. The Japanese exceed at "minimalist art," but minimalist art of any kind - including mantras and symbols - is not easy to do well. Go ask any artist. Reportedly when the Vatican asked Michelangelo for his resume, on the spot he drew a perfect circle. The artists out there know how difficult this is. And yes, he was hired for the job!

So, the terms jumon - a spell, charm, an incantation, a magic word - or mantra - a "tool of the mind" are quite appropriate.

In the ancient Indian arts, which are the progenitors of all of the Asian arts and have greatly influenced all spiritual teachings and religions the world over, the sacred sound/vibrational essence of the Universe has been referred to as the Shabda Brahma, the Nada Brahma, and the Nada Bindu, amongst other sacred names. And there are many Vedic, tantric, and mantric arts (and others) which have been developed for accessing and utilizing this Universal sacred sound. I was initiated by H.H. Sant Rajinder Singh Ji Maharaj into one known as, Surat Shabd Yoga (or, the "yoga of the Light and Sound of God").

CHAPTER TWO: The Seven Jewels of Reiki Overview

The original sound vibration - the Shabda Brahma - which is said to have created our Universe and may still be heard by those sensitive enough vibrating in All, is none other than the sacred Om or Aum. In Sanskrit she is written this way:

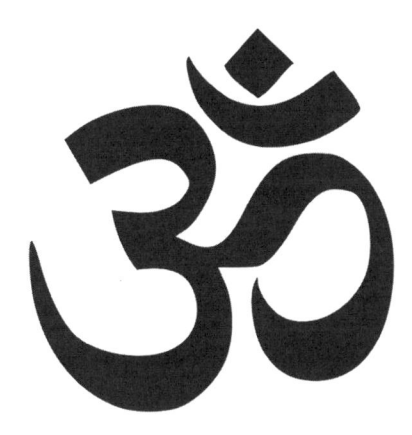

Sanskrit Om

And in Tibetan Uchen script like this:

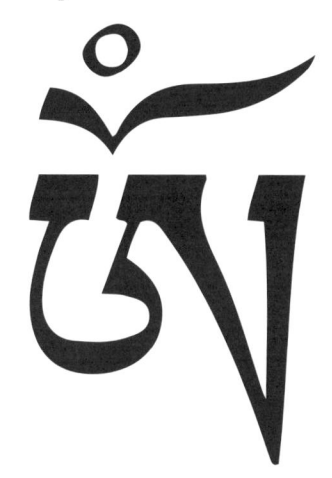

Tibetan Om

The Tibetan calligraphy was modeled upon Sanskrit long ago at the behest of the first Tibetan Buddhist king, and is like a variation of the Sanskrit; a very beautiful one, at that.

Now I'm not presenting myself as an expert on all of this, because I'm not; I am merely sharing some ideas and hopefully opening some minds and eyes, in order for people to do some actual study and research. The use of mantras and symbols did not begin with O-Sensei Usui, in other words. Nor did his mantras and symbols come from outer space, Atlantis, or Tir Na Nog, or anywhere like that. Personally, although I'd love to live in the secret kingdom of Shambhala and play with little Tibetan elves and ride a unicorn - the Usui mantras and symbols didn't come from there, either! There is so much for the interested reiki student to learn regarding the art of reiki and the actual methods and concepts underlying the art. So get out there and study! It's good for the soul. We will still have time for fantasy. And certainly the "real world" and the fantasy/mythic worlds do intersect, I understand this, as only one of my feet is planted "here" - but be aware of where you may be at any moment and where the information is coming from. Ok, I'm off to Middle Earth for a while, a gorgeous Elven Princess awaits...

Now, regarding the jumon which O-Sensei shared with us in the compassionate art of Usui Reiki Ryoho, one of them is an ancient Shamanic symbol of which there are numerous variations of outside of our art (the C.K.R.). The other three are examples of "sacred calligraphy" or "sacred writing." One of these is a simplified version of an ancient Sanskrit seed letter/mantra and symbol (the S.H.K.) known as Hri or Hrim originally. The other two Usui Reiki mantras/symbols are actually kanji - ancient Chinese writing - and the vocalization of these kanji. These are known as H.S.Z.S.N. and D.K.M.

"Sacred writing," "sacred calligraphy," "holy words," "holy script," and "sacred letters" refers to writing or words which have been empowered with the Universal Life Force. They are true "power words" or "power phrases." In this case, the Founder of our art imbued the jumon and shirushi with the power of the Universal Life Force (reiki) so that they would perform and operate as they have been give unto us. Or, we may say that the Universal Life Force operating through him did this.

Now, as to how this process actually happens scientifically speaking is as yet unknown. O-Sensei himself said that his art "rises above modern science." It still does to this day. But that is okay, this is just an example of us making use of natural universal laws which have yet to be discovered. Many things we take for granted and make use of each day are like this. For instance, have you floated above the Earth much lately? No, I didn't think so. Yet how gravity actually is created or works as a universal force is still not fully understood. But it does. We don't need to wait for reiki to be fully understood to make use of and benefit from Her, either. That she is a tremendous positive force for all and is safe and practical is all we need to know. Eventually, the reiki scientists will figure the rest out and a theory will be developed. But why wait when

CHAPTER TWO: The Seven Jewels of Reiki Overview

you can reiki now?

Something else to keep in mind is that without receiving a reiki attunement these jumon (and the shirushi) don't do anything, reiki-wise anyway. They might as well be gibberish. They have no "reiki power" without the reiki attunement. And by the way, this is why they should remain private as "inside information" for reiki practitioners only. So that people don't fool themselves into thinking that because they have read a book and seen the jumon and shirushi that they are reiki practitioners. I have met too many people who have told me this. Remember - no attunement = no reiki!

And worse, they should be private so that unscrupulous people do not try to deceive others into thinking they are great "Reiki Masters" when in fact they have never even taken a class.

This also happens. There was the recent case of the guy who was going around presenting himself like the "Dalai Lama of Reiki" - wearing robes and with a shaved head, but oddly, chain smoking French filter-less cigarettes - and charging very high fees. He caused quite a stir. Then it was found out that he never took a reiki class, he was making it all up and ripping people off... there are too many "snake oil salesmen" out there, be careful.

Thus, no attunement + no training = no reiki teacher!

Intelligence and skill with related arts won't do it either. If I train to be a Buddhist monk, this will not make me a Christian Minister. If I learn how to repair jacuzzis, I may not know how to properly repair a Mercedes Benz. Do you know how many times I have talked to people who have wanted to skip the first reiki class because they may have done some other yoga or meditative-type training? None of these are substitutes for each other. To learn properly we have to humble ourselves and start at the beginning. If we indeed have had good previous training then we will progress a bit faster. But we still need to begin at the beginning.

So, the jumon due to the empowerment via the reiki attunement are one of the key and unique tools of this wonderful and compassionate art. Now let's examine the shirushi (the actual symbols) a bit more.

Shirushi

As we have just seen in the previous discussion, one of the reiki symbols (the C.K.R.) is a simple shamanic symbol or yantra - it is a geometric symbol, not writing. Variations of this symbol outside of the art of reiki are fairly common. In fact, I have learned several "non-traditional" reiki symbols which are similar, as well.

The symbol S.H.K. is not a yantra, however. She is an example of "sacred letters," a variation of the Sanskrit seed letter/mantra Hri or Hrim (kiruku in Japanese). The next two reiki symbols are examples of "sacred writing" or "sacred calligraphy." They are none other than kanji characters, or traditional Chinese writing, which is the foundation of Japanese writing. They are the H.S.Z.S.N. and D.K.M. "symbols."

So technically these last three are not really "symbols" but they are "symbolic," so the word symbol is fine. They work from and upon the principles of symbology.

When we activate and utilize any of these symbols along with their accompanying jumon we are utilizing them as a tool to access various aspects of the Universal Life Force so that healing, transformation, and/or empowerment may be facilitated. Thus, they are indeed "reiki power tools."

The reiki symbols act and gain their power from the "light principle" which pervades all of creation, as the jumon (mantras) gain their power from the vibration/sound principle. And the "Light and Sound Principles" work together, as they are meant to. The "Light of Creation" is no less than All of Creation, all things made manifest. This includes symbols, such as reiki symbols. And all of manifest creation - the Light of Creation - has vibrations (sound) as its essence. And they cannot be separated, not in this Universe anyway.

It may even be understood that all of the untold aspects of manifest Creation, everything - rocks, trees, animals, clouds, stars, the void of space, you and me - are in actuality living "mantras and symbols" of the Divine, imbued with the vibratory and light essence (the "Sound and Light of God"). After all, this is what All is made from. Sound and Light are the very fibers and fabric of Creation, royal garments made of love.

Back to the topic at hand. Thus, we are utilizing the special powers and virtues inherent within these reiki symbols and mantras in order to access the Universal Life Force. The applications are virtually endless, once we get beyond the basic hand positions of reiki. Utilizing the jumon and shirushi always

CHAPTER TWO: The Seven Jewels of Reiki Overview

follows the way of reiki - for the Highest Good of All, Thy Will be Done, not mine. We must check the ego at the door.

Again, what scientifically and theoretically from a scientific viewpoint allows for the symbols and mantras of reiki to work has not yet been discovered. I believe this day will come soon as the scientific community now accepts the "unseen world" and has proven its existence and power and is actively exploring it. But we aren't quite there yet. However, the art of reiki, and the reiki symbols and mantras, do indeed work safely and powerfully, and with compassion, and not as a mere placebo effect. Let me share with you an amusing and enlightening testament to this.

Years ago I participated in a "Nurse Appreciation Week" event at a local hospital. I was there to provide reiki sessions for these noble, hard-working, and compassionate people. Nurses never get enough credit or respect - so thank you Nurses, you guys are real angels - and that goes for you male nurses as well!

Well, at a certain point a middle-aged female doctor sat down to try a reiki session. Good for her. But before I could begin she warned me, "I don't believe in any of this stuff!" Ah, if I had a nickel for every time I have heard this... anyway, I assured her that belief wasn't necessary and began the reiki session. As often happens with very stressed individuals (like virtually all hospital workers, doctors included) during the session she fell sound asleep. I had to kind of hold her up in the chair as I gave her reiki. After about fifteen minutes I gently woke her up, whereupon she looked up at me with a quite startled look on her face and said, "Hey, that stuff really works!" Reiki strikes again. Yes indeed, it does work. Yes, indeed.

"Our method is a spiritual one, it transcends medical science - it is not based on it."

-O-Sensei Mikao Usui

Reiki Chiryo-ho

> "The best methods are those which help the mind and body to resume their inner work of healing."
>
> -Paramahansa Yogananda

Reiki Chiryo-ho refers to the reiki healing methods, or techniques. In other words how one actually applies reiki healing for self or others. These methods proceed from very simple yet highly practical and effective ones, to potentially very esoteric yet no less practical methods.

In general, all of the reiki healing applications of Usui Reiki Ryoho are extremely simple, but in a profound way. They are not as technically complex as the healing methods of many other natural healing arts, such as those utilized in Shiatsu, Thai yoga and Letha yoga body work, pranic healing, or Chinese medicine. Yet again, simple in technical formulation does not mean in any way limited or ineffective in application. Go back and reread some of the examples which I provided of various reiki healing success stories and "reiki miracles." It was the compassionate art of reiki which facilitated these wonderful and blessed healings.

Reiki empowers our own innate healing abilities to work better, which is perhaps the key and most important form of healing we have available to us. This is healing which comes from inside of us, pure and natural. And no strings - or pills, surgical knives, or MRIs - attached! In simple economic terms alone think of the ramifications of this if reiki were to become as universally accepted and widespread as taking a pill was. People think nothing of throwing chemicals down the trap nowadays, to the point that the toxicity from our urine and from flushed pills is even poisoning our drinking water. And please remember, reiki does not nor is not intended to take the place of standard medical practices. This is not the point nor is it the goal. Reiki is part of an individual's total wellness plan and potential, just like hygiene, diet, exercise, nurturing and supportive relationships, and other factors are. Reiki is a living manifestation of the well-known adage, "first, do not harm." So what's to be afraid of? Yes, I can't resist, "have no fear, reiki is here!"

In my book "The Compassionate Touch of Reiki: Healing Concepts, Elements, Methods" we explore the foundational and key reiki healing methods in detail. For now, let's look at some of the important and fundamental concepts of reiki healing. The following diagram outlines the three essential aspects of all forms of healing, whether it be dentistry or reiki. Let's explore it a bit:

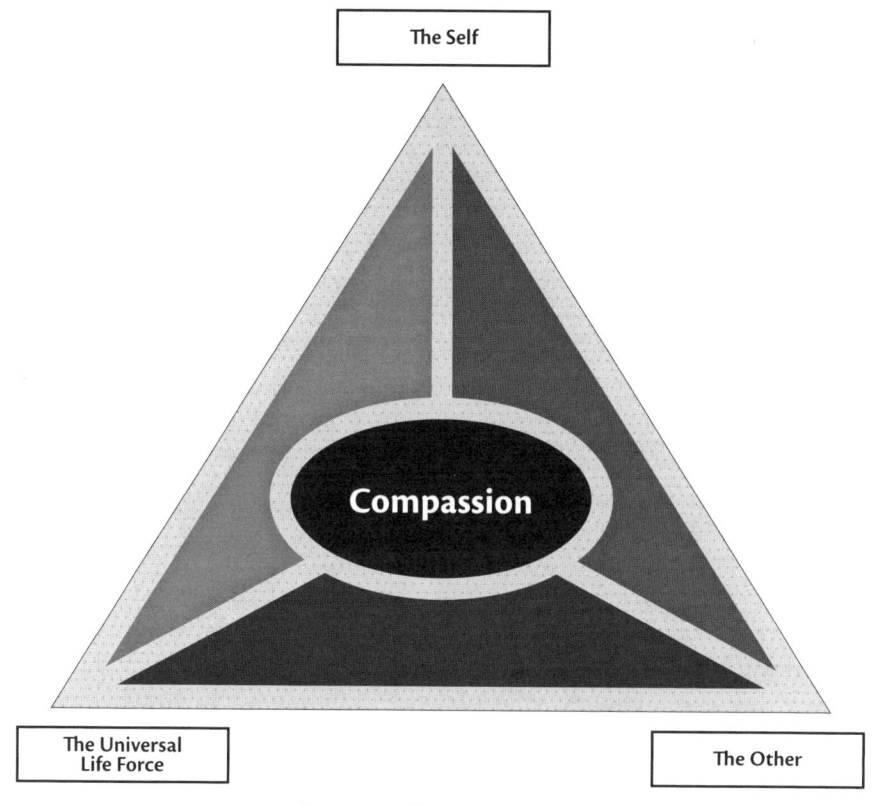

The Healing Pyramid

(Diagram: triangle with "The Self" at top vertex, "The Universal Life Force" at bottom-left vertex, "The Other" at bottom-right vertex, and "Compassion" in the center.)

The Self

The key elements in all forms of healing are our self and compassion. In fact, we may refer to these as the "spark of healing," for they ignite the seeds of healing within for our Highest Good. We can be our own best friend when it comes to health and healing, or our own worst enemy. The choice is up to us, and we do indeed have a choice. And we should choose compassion for ourselves and for all, each and every day.

No matter what we may be facing, no matter how serious the challenge, we can choose to be a positive participant in our own healing process. In one famous example, Dr. Bernie Siegel - facing terminal illness - laughed his way to health, literally. He decided not to worry about it, and watched funny movies and enjoyed his time as best as he could, and with great mirth at that. He is still alive, happy and laughing, to this day.

Truly, it is our emotions and our reactions to our emotions and the negative stress within and around us which is the primary cause of most illness. Think about it - if we are unbalanced within, if we are unharmonious and unhappy within - how can we be healthy? We might as well be a software program infested with viruses bent upon our destruction.

Yet, we all hold the power within us to change this sad situation. The compassionate art and teachings of reiki are one path we can follow to do this- an ideal, simple, yet practical and effective one. And there are other such paths. Being involved in this field for some time now, and reflecting upon my own healing journey, I believe that one of the biggest stumbling blocks to becoming the Captain of our own ship of health and healing is none other than sheer ignorance. In our "modern" culture most of us are not taught that we can - or that we even should - be involved in our own healing process. Healing is viewed as something which comes from "outside" of ourselves and which is beyond our own control. You know, as in, "take two aspirin and call the doctor in the morning." This is the prevailing attitude of modern culture, that healing is completely in the hands of the other, healing exists in a pill, a drug, a surgery, a machine - or some combination of these. In our rush to be modern and in the amazing industrialization and technologization of the past 150 years we have forgotten some of the most important wisdom of our past. This wisdom should not be forsaken or forgotten - the ancient and modern can learn to live together, to the mutual benefit of us all.

When I first heard that it is our emotions that generally make us sick, and that no one could know me better than me - including how I should pursue my own path of healing - I was actually shocked. Like most of us, if I thought about it at all (that's the other thing, we are all taught so well that we don't even contemplate such things, it isn't a regular part of the programming in tv guides) I figured that it was all beyond my control. Health came from my genetics, from the circumstances of my birth, how much money I had, and the like. I had never heard that health actually comes from within, and that we have the keys to healing within ourselves. Yet I contemplated this when I first heard it from my oh-so-wise taiji teacher, and examined the issue within myself and those around me. And I found it to be true. This realization opened my eyes to a whole new world. This same teacher also taught me that "the greatest miracle is a permanent change to a higher state of consciousness." Well, I guess we must call it a miracle then, for now I understand that the attitude with which we live day to day sets the tone for all else. Yes, we must be humble, we must be compassionate, and we must be forgiving.

But we must also learn to develop unshakeable, adamantine self-confidence-

CHAPTER TWO: The Seven Jewels of Reiki Overview

true self-confidence, the kind which only comes from within, from our Soul or Higher Self. Not anything false, prideful, or delusional. The kind of confidence which can only come from learning to value ourselves and to love ourselves, so that we may give ourselves the kind of love which we all deserve- the true love and compassion, which come from the heart and soul. This inner love and self-confidence involves many factors and the path to manifesting it may be as different as each of us is different. Regardless, it begins the same way for us all, with the realization that healing and confidence and loving ourselves is possible. In fact, truly it is how we are meant to live, all of us. Not just the elite, the fortunate ones, or the lucky ones. All human beings deserve this, and that means you do, too.

My very special early reiki teacher, the highly gifted and clairvoyant artist, put it to me this way in my first reiki class with her: "we need to keep open the possibility that one day, just maybe, perhaps, when we are comfortable and ready, at some point in time, that we might be open to being open to the possibility of healing - perhaps, I'm not sure, but just maybe - someday."

Even an intention as tentative as this one will begin to open the window of healing, letting in the Universe's healing rays of sunshine; so that the dusty and gloomy, sick, unbalanced, and diseased areas of ourselves and our lives may begin to brighten - even if it is only in a potential form. Even from this faint intention to heal, the seed within will begin to germinate. Such is the awesome power that our intention combined with the Universal Life Force contains within it, in a latent form just waiting to be activated. Hallelujah for this!

I have come from a far, far place on my path of healing. I was very sick, very beaten down. Yet I always maintained a strong inner core of self-confidence. This was a gift I was born with, to know that I was Soul even from my earliest memories; and which my Saintly Mom nurtured in me despite the chaos and suffering in our lives. I have met individuals who were (and are) much worse than I was, unfortunately - people who told me that they were so far gone that they actually hated themselves and hated life. Imagine living like this, a kind of living hell it must be. Yet I have seen even people like this, with discipline and the help of others - combined with the miraculous healing potential of the Universal Life Force - make complete turnarounds! They live life with a smile on their face each and every day now.

One of my reiki teachers, an extremely gifted and accomplished person who came here from Burma after WWII, works with some of the sickest of the sickest - people who have been wounded terribly in spirit, mind, and body. Imagine having your legs, arms, and genitals blown off in combat, and being blinded as well - yet surviving - surviving to live life flat on your back for decades as essentially a blind, limbless human turtle. May God bless these people who have made such a great sacrifice for their country. Well, my teacher - who is so very gifted and compassionate - is even able to help these poor souls to find a pathway to peace and to healing. God bless him for this gift and God bless them on their journey. Truly it is through our sickness - overcoming and transforming our sickness - that we learn to live as Soul, to live life from the Higher Self, leaving behind the petty and unessential detritus and junk. Thanks be to all of my challenges, for they have taught me the value of life and how to live.

Now, our attitude towards ourselves and our own health and well-being can take many forms. It isn't by any means all esoteric! Thus, nuts and bolts issues like asking questions of healthcare providers and others, educating ourselves about the various facets of our illness and issues are also obviously key. If we don't like the answers we are getting, if it doesn't make sense, or if those who are helping us are not respectful or compassionate - then perhaps we should find others who can do a better job - like looking for a new car mechanic. Yes, we should respect and appreciate experts - but they should also respect and appreciate us - especially when the doc is on vacation in Tuscany dining with the local Maestro. As the Serenity Prayer puts it: God, grant me the serenity to accept the things I cannot change, the courage to change the things I can, and the wisdom to know the difference.

The ultimate, highest form of compassion and self-healing almost seems counter-intuitive, for it involves saying goodbye to the self - the "small self." We must surrender our small self and ego so that we may embrace our Higher Self, Soul, Atman, or Buddha Nature. To do this we dedicate all - including our own selves and self-healing - to the Highest Good of All, Thy Will Be Done, not mine...when we do this truly amazing and miraculous healing can happen, as we will then be living as pure vessels for the Universal Life Force. Thus, as a reiki person, I like to put it this way, "Let go, Let Reiki."

The Universal Life Force

The Universal Life Force (reiki) is another of the key elements of all forms of healing, as the Healing Pyramid illustrates. In fact, combined with our intention - which is the "spark" of healing - it is the "modus operandi" of healing. Whether it be directly or indirectly, consciously or unconsciously - the Universal Life Force is always there offering us support and nurturance, energy and fuel, love and light - as we travel the path of Life.

Of course, in a compassionate healing art such as Usui Reiki Ryoho, this

CHAPTER TWO: The Seven Jewels of Reiki Overview

is evident right from the beginning, as the Universal Life Force is the very "medicine" and the "technology" which empowers the art. But even in forms of healing which are not directly based upon the powers and virtues of reiki, she is still there offering her unseen but undeniable support. For instance, what is it that empowers the dentist's consciousness, mind, and body, so that she may perform her wonderful and much appreciated skills? What gave her life so that she might pursue this vocation? And how did the designers of the tools the dentist utilizes, and the makers of the medications involved, derive the intelligence and inspiration to develop them?

Of course, this is none other than the Universal Life Force! I urge everyone to remember the great Bard's wise verse, "a rose by any other name would smell as sweet." Let's not get lost in linguistic traps.

So, really there is virtually no difference between reiki as Universal Life Force, reiki as healing energy, or the Universal Life Force as the Great Spirit or God. These are merely facets of the same beautiful and mysterious jewel. Can we separate God from God's love? Let us not let our dim human minds and eyes darken Her Light. Reiki as Universal Life Force Healing Energy can never be separated from reiki as Source. Ever. She is indestructible and immutable pure Light, however She may manifest or be perceived. Just as Yin may never be separated from Yang - all there is, is the Dao. Perfect, whole, and complete. Only in our ignorance and delusion do we see "differences" like this. When we view them from Higher Self they vanish. How many angels can fit on the head of a pin? The answer is as many as want to be there... if they are truly God's Angels. Questions like this are stupid and childish.

In the vast, mysterious, emptiness of eternity all there is, is the Ki, the Light. All of the untold and innumerable manifestations which we see and experience of this Eternal Ki are merely facets of Her one brilliance. The terms "reiki" or "Universal Life Force" are ways of talking about this Eternal, one Ki from the viewpoint of this understanding. That is it. Complex systems of ki, ch'i, and prana exist only to help us to learn about and make use of the one, true Ki. Do not let them confuse you, however, into thinking that there are in fact "different kinds of ki." There aren't. All there is, is the Eternal, Great, Bright Light. All the rest is just various shades and colorings and flavorings - the beautiful music and art of Creation.

In Christianity there is the teaching of the Father, the Son, and the Holy Ghost. And first let me say respectfully that I am no Christian scholar, and mean no disrespect to any Christians or Scholars out there. The following are my own observations. Esoterically - in my humble understanding and how I have been taught and come to realize - this means God the Father as Great Spirit - the Universal Life Force of all Creation and beyond all creations; and God the Father as the timeless and eternal which was never born and will never die.

The Son stands for our Soul, or Higher Self, the Atman, or Buddha Nature. The "Son" is indistinguishable from the "Father," being the pure reflection of the "Father" here in Creation, in our universe and dimension. The "Son" exists in all of us, and indeed in all things, all beings, all there is here. Even a tiny pebble contains the spark of the Divine Father.

And the Holy Ghost symbolizes the Universal Life Force as the vivifying power of the "Father" - as in, "And God said, let there be Light, and there was Light." This is the same healing and vivifying and harmonizing power which reiki practitioners are making use of - Holy Ghost Power! Amen to that. Of course, we could also call it "Buddha Power, or reiki, or the Universal Life Force, or the Divine Light. They are all just terms for the same miraculous force.

In reiki terms we may outline this as follows:

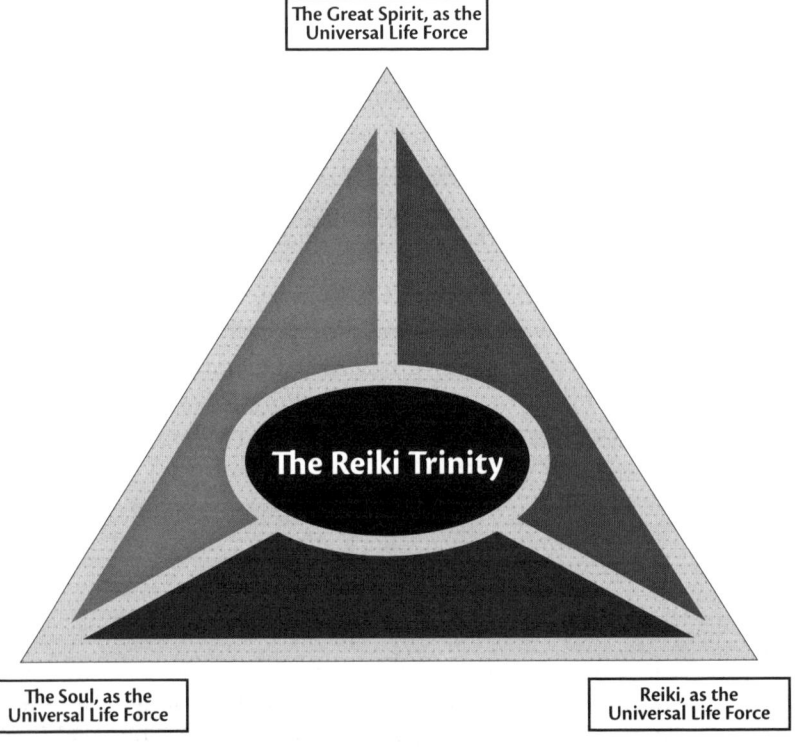

```
                The Great Spirit, as the
                Universal Life Force

                    The Reiki Trinity

   The Soul, as the                    Reiki, as the
   Universal Life Force                Universal Life Force
```

The Reiki Trinity

CHAPTER TWO: The Seven Jewels of Reiki Overview

But remember, this is just a simple formula to help us to understand and work with reiki. In the end all there is, is the Ki - perfect, pure, formless, and eternal. And this Great Ki is Divine Love.

There is much more which could be said about the ramifications of the Reiki Trinity. For now, we will leave it here, understanding that the Universal Life Force is an undeniable and indispensable element of the Healing Pyramid and of all forms of healing.

The Other

The last - but by no means the least - element of the Healing Pyramid is known as the Other. This is generally another person, but it could just as well be any other aspect of Nature - a pet, a tree, a butterfly, a shoe, the clouds, lakes and rivers, the air we breathe - anything may take the role of the other in order to aid and promote healing. All aspects of Nature and the Univers, being imbued with the Universal Life Force, are potential healing agents, sparks, or ignitors and conveyors of healing. The shamans and Spirit Healers of all cultures know this, as did O-Sensei Usui, who taught this as well.

For now we are going to focus on the Other as a person, another person who is assisting us somehow as we walk the healing path.

Even in reiki self-healing the Other plays a vital and prominent role. For instance, someone taught me how to do this and gave me a reiki attunement. My parents conceived me and gave me life, so that I might have the precious opportunity and gift of human life and all that entails - such as learning the compassionate art of reiki.

And obviously, if we are receiving any kind of direct healing or treatment from someone else, then they are performing the vital role of the Other for us. We all depend upon the assistance of others, and in a million ways. In fact, if it wasn't for help from others - along with the Universal Life Force - we wouldn't even be here. Such is the love that the Universe has for us that we are provided with this support. Note that expressing kindness and gratitude to others, and for life in general, are some of the key features of the Gokai, or Reiki Life Concepts. This is as much for our own self-healing as it is for acknowledging the gifts and blessings which others - as well as the Universal Life Force - have bestowed upon us.

This goes for the super-rich, wealthy, elite, and powerful as well. We are all - this includes you folks as well-human beings, equal sons and daughters of the same Universal Life Force. No better, no worse, and no different than anyone else. You are not God, you are not above the laws of Nature. If you were placed alone with all of your billions upon a deserted island, you would suffer like everyone else. And one way or another, death is waiting to tap you on the shoulder someday, the same as he will for us all. So why not join the human race, come back to the family. We love you! Think of the good you could do if you considered yourself a part of the human family and a part of Nature, rather than somehow above them.

Now, unfortunately, in "modern medicine," this one element of the "Healing Pyramid" - the Other - has come to completely dominate the other two, to the point of even denying that one of them exists (the Universal Life Force). Spirituality was even classified as a mental disorder at one time! Talk about power - that sure is one way to promote business - declare everyone else is crazy, and use your political connections to enforce this. Nice!

Well, actually, we reiki practitioners are not delusional or crazed cult fanatics, nor are we psychotic or schizophrenic lost souls. Ah, it's actually almost amusing to see how unbalanced our society has become. For in actuality it is those who deny or denigrate the "unseen world" who are delusional, sick, or confused. Not the other way around. But no worries, with respect for all and compassion, we that are reiki are here to wake everyone up and to play our part in the macro-healing and rebalancing and harmonizing of our society and our planet. And our hands are only full of love and light, not weapons. We love you all. How we got to the point that these two key areas of healing- ourselves and the Universal Life Force - became so trivialized is a fascinating and sad tale. Its principle characters are none other than an unholy trinity known as Politics, Business, and Religion. Like all forms of power and energy, these three can be utilized as forces for good, as tools of healing and transformation dedicated to the Highest Good, or not. When their powers are fused together they become virtually unstoppable - again for good or ill, depending on how they are utilized. But this is a huge and controversial topic best left for another day and a different book.

So, as you can see, the Other, whether in the micro-cosmic realm of self-healing or the macro-cosmic realm of world healing, plays an integral and oh so influential role. May we, in our role as the Other, always seek to assist and lead others with compassion and with love. And each and every day, as this is the reiki way.

Another important aspect of the Healing Pyramid is that none of these three elements can be separated; they exist in a relationship to each other. Each of these aspects are reflections of each other. Even in such a rare instance as

CHAPTER TWO: The Seven Jewels of Reiki Overview

O-Sensei Usui's "Divine Attunement" upon Mt. Kurarna all of these elements are there. And the compassionate art of Usui Reiki Ryoho serves as a powerful and dynamic example of all elements of the Healing Pyramid - when one experiences reiki first hand it cannot be denied or explained away.

This art is such a gentle, respectful, pure, yet potentially powerful and life-changing art. It is so wonderful that it operates safely, virtually above and beyond the consciousness of the one utilizing or receiving Her, It is as pure and ego-less a healing art that is possible for us while we exist in a human body - a great, most high and beautiful, loving and wise - yet practical and effective - gift of Nature and the Universe.

We will be exploring the fundamental reiki healing methods in detail in the next book in this series, The Compassionate Touch of Reiki: Healing Concepts, Elements, Methods. Here in this book we have been exploring the foundations of reiki, reiki concepts and principles, what is reiki, what makes this art unique, and all related. In book two we will be exploring the essential reiki concepts and elements; as well as the key meditation, reiki-ko methods, and reiki healing methods for self and others.

The reiki healing methods (reiki chiryo-ho) follow the outline presented earlier in the first chapter, the "Scope of Reiki Healing." The art of reiki is what is known as a High - Internal healing system. She uses no medicines/herbs and no tools - other than those which Nature and the Universe has already provided us with. The reiki energy is the "medicine" and we are Her vessel, or "tool." How beautiful is that? And even better, reiki can enhance and augment all other forms of healing, as she is none other than the pure essence of healing personified.

The reiki healing methods, as we shall see, proceed from simple, light hand placement techniques, routines, and methods for self and others; to more esoteric methods making use of the reiki and of the jumon and shirushi in various ways. But esoteric does not mean less practical, just more subtle.

All in all, Usui Reiki Ryoho is a simple, non- technical, non-dogmatic -yet highly diverse and practical - healing method that is appropriate for all people. She is compassionate yet potentially very powerful as well, a great blessing. As I sit and write this it is actually the anniversary of O-Sensei's birthday. What an appropriate time to thank him for sharing this gift with the world. Gassho, Namaste, amen.

Summary of Chapter Two:

- The Seven Jewels of Reiki are the main elements of the art of Usui Reiki Ryoho
- Gassho symbolizes the meditative intent and methods of the art, and is the core and central pillar of the entire system
- Reiju refers to the "reiki gift," or reiki attunement, and is how one acquires reiki healing ability (the only way)
- Gokai refers to the Reiki Life Principles, which were given to us by the Founder, O-Sensei Mikao Usui
- Reiki-ko is the reiki sub-art of specialized reiki meditations, breathing exercises, and energy exercises
- Jumon refers to the reiki "mantras"
- Shirushi refers to the reiki "symbols"
- Reiki chiryo-ho are the actual reiki healing methods, for self and others
- Usui Reiki Ryoho is a "High-Internal" healing system based on compassion and the blessings of the Universal Life Force
- The Healing Pyramid illustrates the three interconnected elements of all forms of healing, including reiki
- The Reiki Trinity are the three virtually identical and indistinguishable aspects of the Universal Life Force; we may perceive them as distinct, but they are really reflections of the same One Brilliance, the same Eternal Universal Flame

Appendix: Reiki Historical Documents

The following are four important historical documents regarding the history and practice of the compassionate art of reiki. Many thanks to Sensei James Deacon for allowing me to share his translations and documents which he makes available on his wonderful website, www.aetw.org. In my opinion this is the very top online resource for quality information on all aspects of reiki and Usui Reiki Ryoho.

The first document is the translation of the Usui Memorial. It speaks of O-Sensei's life and achievements as the Founder of his art, what we now refer to as Usui Reiki Ryoho. The memorial was erected in February, 1927 and is at the Jodo Shu Saihoji Temple in Tokyo, Japan...Jodo Shu is of the Buddhist "Pure Land" school.

Next is a translation of an actual interview with O-Sensei Usui which is part of a manual which was passed out to Japanese reiki students in Japan, the Reiki Ryoho Hikkei (Reiki Treatment Companion). What is shared here is the Q & A section with O-Sensei, most fascinating and invaluable.

Next are copies of two newspaper interviews with Rev. Hawayo Takata, the heir of Shihan Hayashi and person responsible for bringing the art to the world. Mahalo a nui Rev. Takata!

Reiho Choso Usui Sensei Kudoku No Hi

Memorial of the Benevolence of Usui Sensei, founder of Reiho (Spiritual Method)

English Version, Copyright © 2003 **James Deacon**
Translation (especially for AETW.org) by **Jiro Kozuki**

That which one attains within, as a result of disciplined study and training, is called Virtue, and that which can be offered to others by teaching, and methods of salvation is called Distinguished Service. Only the person of high merit and great virtue can be called a great founding teacher. Sages, philosophers, and brilliant men of old and the founders of new teachings and new religions were all like that. Usui Sensei can be counted among them. Usui Sensei developed the method that would improve mind and body by using the universal power. Having heard of his reputation, countless people from all over gathered and asked him to teach them the great way of the Spiritual Method, and to heal them.

His common name was Mikao and his other name was Gyoho (Kyoho). He was born in the village of Taniai in the Yamagata district of Gifu prefecture. His ancestor's name is Tsunetane Chiba. His father's name was Taneuji, and was commonly called Uzaemon. His mother's family name was Kawai.

Sensei was born in the first year of the Keio period, called Keio Gunnen (1865), on August 15th. He was a talented and hard working student; his ability was far superior to his fellows. When he had grown up, he travelled to Europe, America and China to study. He wanted to be successful in life, but couldn't achieve it. He worked hard but often he was unlucky and in need. However he didn't give up and he disciplined himself to study more and more.

One day he went to Kurama Yama to undergo rigourous spiritual discipline. On the beginning of the 21st day, suddenly he felt a large Reiki over his head. He attained an enlightenment and at that moment he comprehended the Spiritual Method. When he first used it on himself, it produced beneficial results immediately. After that, he tried it on his family. Since it was effective, he decided it was much better to share it with the public than to keep this knowledge solely for his own family. He opened a training centre in Harajuku, Aoyama, Tokyo to teach and practice the Spiritual Method in April of the 11th year of the Taisho period (1922). Many people came from far and wide and asked for the guidance and therapy, and even lined up outside of the building.

In September of the twelfth year of the Taisho period (1923), there was a devastating earthquake. Everywhere there were groans of pain from the injured. Usui Sensei felt pity for the people, and took the Spiritual Method into the devastated city and used its healing powers on the survivors, curing and saving innumerable people. This is just a broad outline of his relief activities during such an emergency.

Later on, his training centre became too small. In February of the 14th year of Taisho (1925 A.D.) he moved to a new training centre in Nakano, outside Tokyo. Due to his increased fame he was often invited to many places. Sensei, accepting the invitations, went to Kure and then to Hiroshima and Saga, and reached Fukuyama. It was during his stay in Fukuyama that unexpectedly he became ill and died, aged 62*. It was March 9 of the 15th year of Taisho (1926 A.D.) [*NOTE: According to the dates given, Usui Sensei would have actually been 60 at the time of his death. However, apparently there is an ancient Japanese tradition that a child is considered to be 'one' at birth, and is seen as being a year older at each new year, rather than the birthday that falls in that year?? An alternative explanation for the discrepancy could have something to do with the fact that, at the time of Usui-sensei's birth, Japan used a different calendrical system. The change over to the 'western' system in 1873 may have led to mistakes in the recording of exact dates of events in the immediately preceding years??] His wife was named Sadako, from the Suzuki family. A boy and a girl were born. The boy's name was Fuji who carried on the Usui family after his father's death. Sensei was mild, gentle and modest by nature and he never behaved ostentatiously. His was physically big and strong. He always had a contented smile. However, in the face of adversity, he sought a solution with determination and patience. He had many talents and liked to read, and his knowledge of history, medicine, psychology, divination, incantation, physiognomy and Buddhist scriptures was great.

On reflection, the Spiritual Method not only cures diseases, but also balances the spirit and makes the body healthy using innate healing abilities, and so, helps achieve happiness.

So, when it comes to teaching, first let the student understand the Meiji Emperor's admonitions; and let them chant the Five Precepts mornings and evenings, and keep them in mind:

Firstly: Don't get angry today, Secondly: Don't worry today, Thirdly: Be grateful today, Fourthly: Work diligently today , Fifthly: Be kind to others today.

These are truly great teachings for cultivation and discipline in keeping with those great teachings of the ancient sages and the wisemen. Sensei named these teachings 'the Secret Method of Inviting Blessings' and 'the Spiritual Med-

APPENDIX

icine to cure many diseases'. Notice the outstanding features of the teachings. Furthermore, when it comes to teaching, it should be as simple as possible and not difficult to understand. It is important to start from a place close to you. Another noted feature is that while sitting in silent meditation with your hands held in prayer and reciting the Five Precepts, a pure and healthy mind will be cultivated. Its true value is in daily practice. This is the reason why the Spiritual Method became so popular.

Recently the state of the world has altered and peoples' thoughts have changed a great deal. Hopefully, the spread of this Spiritual Method will be of great help to people who have a confused mind or who do not have morality. Surely it is not only of benefit in curing chronic diseases and lingering complaints?

The number of students of Sensei's teaching is already over 2,000. Among them, senior students who remained in Tokyo are maintaining Sensei's training centre, and others in different provinces also are trying to spread the Spiritual Method as much as possible. Although Sensei died, the Spiritual Method will continue to spread far and wide. Ah, what a great thing Sensei has done, to have shared this Spiritual Method with the people out there after having been enlightened within!

Lately, many students came together and decided to erect this memorial in the graveyard at Saihoji Temple in the Toyotama district to honour his benevolence, and to spread the Spiritual Method to the people in the future. I was asked to write these words. As I deeply appreciate his work and am pleased with the very friendly teacher-disciple relationships among fellow students, I could not refuse the request, and I wrote this summary in the hope that people will be reminded to look up to him with reverence.

Composed by: Masayuki Okada, Doctor of Literature - subordinate 3rd rank, 3rd Order of Merit.

Calligraphy by: Navy Rear Admiral Juzaburo Ushida - subordinate 4th rank, 3rd Order of Merit, distinguished service 4th class.

February, the 2nd year of Showa (1927 A.D.)

Questions & Answers From The "Hikkei"

Copyright © 2005 James Deacon

The '*Hikkei* - that is: the *Reiki Ryoho Hikkei* (Reiki Treatment Companion) is a 68 page manual, said to be given to Level 1 (Shoden) students of the Usui Reiki Ryoho Gakkai.

The 'Hikkei is comprised of: an introductory explanation & a Reiki Q & A section (supposedly in Usui Sensei's own words), a healing guide (Ryoho Shishin), & *Gyosei* - waka poetry penned by the Emperor Meiji.

We are told that the 'Hikkei' was compiled in the 1970's by Kimiko Koyama, sixth *kaicho* (president / chairman) of the Usui Reiki Ryoho Gakkai.

What follows is a translation of the Q & A section.

"Why I make these teachings public"
- an explanation by the founder Mikao Usui
[English Version, Copyright © 2004/5 James Deacon]

It's an old tradition that if someone discovers a secret art, they keep it within the family to secure a future for their heirs and descendants. It is not shared with others.

But this is an old-fashioned custom from the old century. In this modern era human happiness is based on living and working together and a desire for social development. For this reason, I wont allow it to just be kept within the family.

Our method is something completely original, there is nothing like it in the whole world. Therefore, I want to share it with the public for the benefit of all humanity. Everyone has the potential to receive the spiritual gift, uniting body and soul, a divine blessing.

Our method is an original one, based on the spiritual power of the universe. By this power, first a person becomes healthy, then the mind becomes calm and life becomes more joyous.

Nowadays, we need to restructure and improve our lives within and without, that we may free our fellow beings from emotional and physical suffering.

This is why I make these teachings public.

What is Usui Reiki Ryoho?

Gratefully we have received the Meiji Emperor's precepts. That humanity may discover its proper path, we must live according to these precepts. We must learn to improve body and heart-spirit [kokoro]. First we heal the heart-spirit, then we make the body healthy. When the heart-spirit finds the healthy, righteous path, the body will automatically become healthy. Thus heart-spirit and body are in harmony and our life is joyous and peaceful. We heal of ourselves and others and deepen the happiness of ourselves and others. This is the aim of Usui Reiki Ryoho.

Is Usui Reiki Ryoho like hypnosis, **kiai jutsu** treatment*, **shinko ryoho** (religious healing) *or similar, just under a different name?*
[* Using the voice to express and direct concentrated ki]

No, no. There is no similarity to any of these methods. After many years of rigorous spiritual discipline, I discovered a spiritual secret: a method of freeing the body and soul [rei].

Is it a spiritual healing method [shinrei ryoho]?

Yes, you could call it that. But it is also a physical healing method as ki and light radiate from the body of the practitioner - particularly from their hands, eyes and mouth. So if they focus the eyes, breathe on, or stroke the affected area, pain such as toothache, headache, neuralgia, colic, stomach-ache, cuts, bruises, burns, etc. will be gone. However, chronic disorders are not that easy to treat - they take time. But even one treatment will bring signs of improvement. How can medical science explain this phenomenon? Well, the reality is more impressive than fiction. If you observed the results for yourself you would agree. Even those who don›t want to believe cannot ignore the results.

Is belief in Usui Reiki Ryoho necessary for healing to be effective?

No, it isn't a psychological method like psychotherapy or hypnosis. As it is not based on suggestion, faith and acquiescence are not required. It doesn't matter if a person doubts or flatly refuses to believe in it. For example, it works just as well with small children and those who are seriously ill and unconscious. Perhaps one in ten has faith in our method before treatment, but after that first treatment most people feel the benefits and then their faith develops.

What can be cured by Usui Reiki Ryoho?

All disorders, whether psychological or organic in origin can be treated by

APPENDIX

this method.

Does Usui Reiki Ryoho only heal physical illnesses/diseases?

No, it not only heals physical problems - it can also heal bad habits and psychological disorders such as despair, weakness (of character), timidity, indecisiveness and nervousness. Through this method the heart-spirit identifies with the divine nature and we desire to heal others. This is how we achieve happiness.

How does Usui Reiki Ryoho work?

I did not receive this method from anyone else. Nor did I train or study to develop supernatural powers. While fasting, I had a mystical experience - I felt an intense energy - and with it, the realization that I had received the spiritual gift of healing. So, even though I am the founder of this method, I find it hard to explain it clearly. Physicians and scholars have been researching such phenomena, but as yet, it has been difficult to reach a scientific explanation. One day, there will be a scientific explanation.

Does Usui Reiki Ryoho use medicines and are there any side effects?

It does not use medicines or medical equipment. Only focussing the eyes, blowing, laying on of hands, tapping, and stroking. This is how it heals.

In order to use Usui Reiki Ryoho does one need medical knowledge?

Our method is a spiritual one, it transcends medical science - it is not based on it. The desired effect is achieved by focussing with the eyes, blowing on, touching or stroking the affected area. For example, for brain problems, give treatment to the head; for stomach problems, the stomach; for eye disorders, treat the eyes. There is no need for bitter medicines or burning *moxa* treatments, yet within a short time you will be returned to health. This is why our spiritual method [*reiho*] is quite original.

What do well-known medical practitioners think about it?

The well-known medical practitioners seem fair in their assessments. Nowadays, western-style physicians are very critical of over-prescription of medicines.

Dr Sen Nagai from Teikoku Medical University said: "As physicians, we know how to diagnose, record and understand illness, but we don't really know how to treat it".

DR Kondo said:"It is arrogant to claim that medical science has made great progress, as it fails to address the psychological/spiritual aspect of the patient. This is its biggest shortcoming."

DR Hara said:"It is wrong to treat humans, possessing spiritual wisdom, like animals. It is my belief that in the future we can expect a great transformation in the therapeutic field."

DR Kuga said:"The fact is that therapists who are not trained physicians have achieved higher levels of success than medical doctors because their therapies take into account the character and personal symptoms of the patient and utilize many different methods of treatment. It would be very narrow-minded for the medical establishment to blindly reject these therapists or attempt to impede their practice." *(from the medical journal: 'Japanese Medical News')*

Doctors and pharmacists often recognize this fact and come to receive training (in our method).

What does the government think?

On February 6th 1922, Parliamentary Representative Teiji Matsushita, asked the Budget Committee about the government's position on therapists practicing spiritual and psycho-therapy without a medical practitioner's licence.

Mr Ushio, a Committee member replied "Little more than a decade ago hypnosis and similar practices were considered demonic, but nowadays, after proper research these practices are effectively used to treat psychiatric patients. It is difficult to try to solve all human problems with medical science. Physicians adhere to scientific medical practices in order to treat disease. The Medical Faculty does not consider touch therapy or electro-therapy to be medical practices."

This is why our method is subject to neither those regulations governing medical practitioners, nor those governing acupuncture or *moxa*heat therapy.

Surely such healing abilities only come to those who are spiritually evolved, rather than through training?

No, not so. Every living, breathing being possesses the spiritual ability to heal. This is true of plants, animals, fish and insects, but it is humans - the culmination of creation - who possess the greatest power. Our method is a practical manifestation of this power.

Can anyone receive initiation into Usui Reiki Ryoho?

Of course. Men and women, old or young, educated and uneducated - anyone with natural (moral?) sense can certainly receive the ability in a short time to treat themselves and others.

I have taught more than a thousand people and not one has failed to have the desired result. Even those who have only learned *shoden* have gained the ability to treat illnesses.

Thinking about it it seems strange that we can gain the ability to heal in such a short time - something so difficult for people to do. But this is the thing about our spiritual method - that we can learn to do something so difficult in a simple way.

So, I can heal other people with it, but can I also heal myself?

If we can't heal our own disorders, how could we heal others?

How can I receive the second degree (Okuden) - what does it involve?

Okuden consists of several methods - hatsu rei ho; patting, stroking and pressing hands; distance treatment; healing of habits/propensities; etc. We will give *okuden* to enthusiastic *shoden* students who bring good results, are of good character, and behave properly.

Is there still more beyond Okuden?

Yes, there is Shinpiden level. [pron: '*shim-pe-den*']

Mrs Takata and Reiki Power

by Patsy Matsuura
(Staff Writer, the Honolulu Advertiser)
(February 25, 1974)

Reprinted from www.aetw.org

There's power in them palms. Mrs. Hawayo Takata, the only Reiki master in Hawaii, claims to possess the key to energy. No, it's not a key to ease the energy crisis. "It's a cosmic energy to heal the ill", said the youthful-looking 73-year-old matron. "Reiki, which is applied by hand, goes to the cause and effect. When the cause is removed there will be no effect. It is not associated with any visible material being. It's an unseen spiritual power that radiates vibration and lifts one into harmony. This power is incomprehensible to man, yet every single living being is receiving its blessings.

"I believe there is only one Supreme Being - the Absolute Infinite - a dynamic force that governs the world and the universe. It is a universal force from the divine spirit and is available to anyone interested in learning the art of healing. "Reiki helps attain health, happiness and security which leads to the road of longevity."

Born in 1900 in Hanamaulu, Kauai, to the late Mr. and Mrs. Otogoro Kawamura, immigrants from Japan, Mrs. Takata was named "Hawayo" after the Territory of Hawaii. Immediately after her birth, she said the attending midwife held her up, patted her head three times and predicted she would be a success.

The Kawamuras envisioned a long and useful life for Hawayo since her older sister, Kawayo, who was named after Kauai, had died at an early age. They wanted their younger daughter to be worthy of her name for to them she "represented" the Hawaiian Islands.

As foreseen by her parents, Mrs. Takata reached her "heights". From her 10th-floor suite in the McCully district, she viewed the city with an air of fulfilment. When I finally caught up with her, she had already played nine holes of golf and had given Reiki treatments to several patients. "I've been playing golf every morning for nearly 30 years", she declared. "And I don't ride the cart either - I walk. It's good exercise. Before coming to Honolulu I lived on Hawaii for several years because I wasn't satisfied until I had been on the Big Island. I bought some land, built a home, and remained there for several years".

Recalling her past, Mrs. Takata said she wasn't always a picture of health. In 1935 when she was 35, she suffered from several illnesses, the major one being asthma. She entered a hospital in Tokyo for an operation. While there she heard about Reiki and decided to try it first. While under the care of Reiki master Chujiro Hayashi for four months, Mrs. Takata recovered. She remained in Japan for one year and mastered the art of healing. During the 39 years of practising Reiki in Hawaii, she acquired clients from all corners of the globe, including Barbara Hutton and Doris Duke. The latter broke her wrist in 1957 and was treated by Mrs. Takata. She became a pupil. "Reiki is available to anyone who seeks it," said Mrs. Takata.

"When a student is ready to accept it, he is shown the way. With the first contact or initiation the hands radiate vibration to the ailing spot. If there is pain, it registers on your fingertips and palms. The ailment disappears when the body responds to the treatment.

"A proper diet enhances the treatments. Vegetables and fruits are excellent foods, but never eat when you're worried. Go to the table only when you're in a pleasant mood. We came into this world for a purpose so we must have health and happiness to achieve our goals. I owe my good fortune to my late husband, Saichi, who was a guiding light until his death in 1930."

Mrs. Takata said she plans to teach Reiki until December 24, 1977, and if she can find a successor she hopes to build a Reiki Center on the three acres of land she owns in Olaa, near Kurtistown, Hawaii. In the event she cannot find a capable replacement, the lot will be turned over to the county of Honolulu.

Meanwhile, she is busy writing a book, "Look Younger, Feel Stronger, and a Way to Longevity" [11] and lecturing at the University of Hawaii.

This spring she will give lectures and lessons on the Mainland, and this summer she had been invited to Indonesia to take part in a five-day festival in the art of healing, sponsored by the Indonesian government.

---

11   This book, it seems was never published

An Interview With Takata-Sensei, May 17, 1975

Mrs. Takata Opens Minds To 'Reiki'

by Vera Graham

(printed in 'The Times', San Mateo, California)

Reprinted from www.aetwa.org

Reiki?

What is Reiki?

Mrs. Hawayo (which means Hawaii) Takata, 74, of Hawaii, the master of Reiki, explains: "Reiki means Universal Life Energy." It is not a religion.

She adds, "It was explained to me this way: 'Here is the great space which surrounds us -- the Universe. There is endless and enormous energy. It is universal. ..Its ultimate source is the Creator. It can stem from the sun, or moon, or stars; that science cannot prove, or tell us, yet. It is a limitless force. It is the source of energy that makes the plants grow... the birds fly.

When a human being has pain, problems, he or she can draw from it. It is an ethereal source, a wave length of great power which can revitalise; restore harmony..."

Mrs. Takata adds in her word, "It is Nature. It is God, the power He makes available to His children who seek it. In Japanese, this is Reiki (Pronounced Ray-Kee).

Sceptics may quit now.

It is interesting to note, however, that Mrs. Takata points out the American Medical Association of Hawaii permits Reiki treatments in hospitals, whenever requested by a patient.

Mrs. Takata will teach Reiki at the University of Hawaii this winter, for which she has a signed contract.

She is living proof that something is very right. At age 74, she plays nine holes of golf daily when at home, and participates in 18-hole tournaments.

She is tiny - and mighty! Projecting tranquillity and quiet strength and power.

She was not always so.

Mrs. Takata recalls when she was 29, her husband died. She was left penniless with two small daughters to rear.

"They alone kept me from suicide," she recalls. "I would look at their small faces as they slept peacefully. I knew I could not do that to them. I was their mother and their father.

"By the time I was 35, I had all kinds of ailments: appendicitis, a benign tumour, gallstones. And to top it, I had asthma, so could not undergo an operation requiring anaesthetic."

"I went down to 97 pounds. Over a period of seven years, I was further emotionally devastated. One dear member of my family died each year.

"I was a church-going woman, and have always believed in God. One day, I meditated, and finally said, "God, I am up against the wall! Help Me!", I said to myself. "If God hears, He will help." As far as I am concerned, that is what happened.

"I heard a voice. Today, we call that clairaudience. I didn't know anything about that in 1935...I heard a voice speak after I complained so bitterly. I felt all alone in the world; as if I alone had all the suffering, burdens, poverty. I had said, "Why am I poor? Why do I have such illness....pain? Why do I have all the sorrows?"

"The voice which replied was loud and clear. It spoke three times. It said, "Number One: Get rid of all your illness.' Just like that! "You will find health, happiness, and security."

"I couldn't believe my ears until I heard the same message three times.

"Within twenty one days, I was on a boat to Tokyo, hoping to find help there. I went to the Maeda Orthopaedic Hospital in the district of Akasaka in Tokyo. That is the finest district in the heart of Tokyo near the Royal Palace. The hospital was named after my friend, Dr. T. Maeda, whom I went to see."

Mrs. Takata says that when Dr. Maeda saw her, she had gone down to 97 pounds. He shook his head, and said she would have to build up her strength before any thought of surgery.

She and her two small daughters stayed at the hospital.

Before continuing with her story, Mrs. Takata explains that Reiki is spoken of

APPENDIX

in the ancient history of Japan, and in the Buddhist Sutras, the sacred writings refer to it. Reiki goes back at least 2,500 years. Its mystery, Mrs. Takata says, was unravelled by Dr. Mikao Usui in the late eighteenth century.

After twenty-one days in the hospital, Mrs. Takata was ready for surgery. She was on the operating table, she recalls, being prepared, when suddenly she again heard the commanding voice.

This time, it said, "Do not have the operation. It is not necessary." Mrs. Takata said she pinched herself, to make sure she was both conscious and sane.

Thrice she heard the admonition, and suddenly got off the operating table and stood on the floor, causing endless consternation among the nurses.

Dr. Maeda came in to inquire. She told him she was not afraid of dying, but wanted to know if there was any other treatment. Dr. Maeda asked how long she would stay in Japan. When she answered, two years, he told the nurses to dress her, and to call his sister, Mrs. Shimura, who was then the hospital dietician.

Mrs. Takata later learned that Mrs. Shimura had, some years previously, been in a coma, dying of dysentery, when a schoolmate of her daughter pleaded with her to seek help for her mother, from the Reiki Master, Dr. Chijuro Hayashi. She did so, and to everyone's amazement, Mrs. Shimura came out of the coma and began to recover.

Mrs. Shimura took her to Dr. Hayashi's offices. "Two of his practitioners worked on me," she recalls. "One on the eyes, head, sinus, thyroid, thymus glands. The other, on the rest of the body. I can best describe it as it is referred to in the Bible: the laying on of hands".

The Maeda Hospital is where they checked and confirmed my progress.

"I am a very curious woman. I said to myself, 'I am going to investigate how they are doing this. What makes me feel first the warmth than actual heat emanating from their hands? I looked under the table, at the ceiling, everywhere. I could find no cords or instruments.

Then I thought, "Aha!, they have a battery hidden in their sleeves." Dr. Hayashi's assistants wore the Japanese kimono with the long sleeves, which have pockets. They worked silently. There was no talking."

"My moment came. When I was being treated, I suddenly grabbed the practitioner by the pocket.

"He was startled, but, thinking I needed some Kleenex, thoughtfully handed me some. I said, "No! I want to see the machine in your pocket." He burst into uncontrolled laughter. Dr. Hayashi came in to see what the commotion was about, and was told.

"...He smiled and shook his head," Mrs. Takata recalls. He proceeded to give her the explanation of a Universal Life Force. He said, "Whenever you feel the contact, all I know is that I have reached this great Universal Life Force, and it comes through me to you - these (he held up his hands) - are the electrodes ....That force begins to revitalise and restore the balance of your entire system."

Mrs. Takata nodded, "Yes," in answer to a query, "Can Reiki help a person who is sincere in a desire to stop drinking to excess, smoking, to lose or gain weight, establish a normal balance of good health?"

In time, Mrs. Takata became convinced that she, too, should learn more and became a student of Dr. Hayashi. She spent months, and was sent into the field to help others. Unbeknownst to her, they made full reports back to Dr. Hayashi. "I passed my examinations perfectly."

Besides the treatments, she adds, there was a matter of special diets, some including sunflower seeds, red beet juice, grapefruit, almonds....

"I speak with confidence about this" Mrs. Takata notes, "but it should be understood I do not speak as 'I... I... I...', I speak because it is of God's power. He is the one who makes it available to us. Who doubts God?..."

Mrs. Takata is the only teacher of the Usui system of Reiki in the world today and is recognized as its master.

APPENDIX

Author's Biography

Michael Fuchs is a life-long reader and writer, enjoying many genres of literature, fiction, and non-fiction; as well as movies and television and the arts in general. A child of amazing artists, he was raised in an artistic environment which encouraged his creativity from birth. He has had editorials and articles published in magazines, such as: Massage Magazine, Tai Chi, Qi: The Journal of Eastern Health and Fitness, and The Empty Vessel. He has been featured on t.v., radio, and in newspapers and magazines numerous times. Sifu Mike is also the author of "The Shaolin Butterfly Style- Art of Transformation" and "The Compassionate Touch of Reiki: Healing Concepts, Elements, Methods."

Mike is a Sifu (Master Teacher) and Instructor in the arts of Shaolin Five Form Fist Kung Fu, Taiji, Kali, Reiki, Qigong, Min Zin and Meditation. He is the former owner and Chief Instructor of the White Lotus Martial Arts Center (est. 1977) and currently leads Butterfly Martial and Healing Arts. Sifu Mike is honored to be the Connecticut State Director for the International Chinese Boxing Association. He has been elected by his peers in the arts into elite Halls of Fame, including the Action Martial Arts Hall of Honors, The Master's Hall of Fame, and the World Karate Union "Lifetime Achievement Award," amongst others.

Sifu Mike has been blessed to learn Reiki Healing Arts and related methods of Min Zin, QiGong, and Meditation from some of the most elite and renowned teachers of these arts. He has also received shaktipata, darshan, satsang, inititian and meditation instruction from famous world level spiritual leaders, such as: Sant Rajinder Singh ji Maharaj, Shri Anandi Ma, Mirabai Devi, Gen Sherab Kelsang, Namadeva Thomas Ashley-Farrand, and Self Realization Fellowship.

Reiki, Taiji, and Martial Arts teachers include: famous living legend, Dr. Maung Gyi; Susane Grasso and Pat Warren (two of the pioneering reiki teachers in the Northeast, USA); Living Treasure Fu Shu Yun; 5 Form Fist Shaolin Headmaster Tao Chi Li; Tuhon Leo T. Gaje; Daoist Lineage Holder Prof. Chung Jie; Sifu Manfred Steiner; Master Wang Hai Jun; Sifu H.K. Chan; Tuhon Bill McGrath; and various others.

Sifu Mike has led Reiki Healing Art programs in the Connecticut State

Prison System and taught Reiki Certification Classes in the Connecticut State Community College System for about ten years. He was also part of the first class of professionally credentialed Integrative Medicine Consultants in the state of CT, via St. Francis Hospital and Medical System (late 1990s), and has led and taught numerous taiji, martial arts, and reiki healing arts multi-day retreats, workshops, seminars and other special events. Sifu Mike has had success integrating his arts of Reiki, Taiji, QiGong, Meditation and Min Zin with traditional medical/healthcare for many special needs groups for close to thirty years now. This includes the Arthritis Foundation, MS Society, Seniors, Prison Populations, Acute Care Rehabilitation and Psychiatric Settings, inner city youth, Spiritual and Religious Retreat settings, in the hospital and medical system/ setting, and others. Recently he has led programs on Reiki and Taiji for the Connecticut Brain Injury Alliance and Project Genesis, and is a Certified Brain Injury Specialist.

Sifu Mike has had success in the martial arts tourney scene as well, both as a trainer and competitor. He trained an extreme full contact weapons fighter who competed in The Gathering of the Pack (Dog Brothers), this young man went undefeated and credited Sifu Mike's training for his success. Later in life Sifu Mike also attended multiple national and world martial art tourneys and had excellent success, such as receiving scores of 10, 10, and 9.9 for his performance of Butterfly/ Yang style taiji at the well-known Ocean State Grand Nationals in 2013 (he was penalized for going over the time limit and finished 3rd), amongst other similar results at national and world tourneys.